Girl,
GET
READY
TO LOSE
THE
DAMN
WEIGHT!

Girl,
GET
READY
TO LOSE
THE
DAMN

WEIGHT!

DR. JADA
MOORE-RUFFIN

publish
y⊕ur gift

GIRL, GET READY TO LOSE THE DAMN WEIGHT!
Copyright © 2021 Jada Moore-Ruffin
All rights reserved.

Published by Publish Your Gift®
An imprint of Purposely Created Publishing Group, LLC

Printed in the United States of America

ISBN: 978-1-64484-307-9 (print)
ISBN: 978-1-64484-308-6 (ebook)

Special discounts are available on bulk quantity purchases by book clubs, associations and special interest groups. For details email: sales@publishyourgift.com or call (888) 949-6228.

For information log on to www.PublishYourGift.com

"Everything we do of substance we do in community with others. I dedicate this book to every person I have ever met on this journey called life, from those closest to me to every stranger with whom I have ever shared a glance, a smile, a word, or a hug. You are my community, you are my inspiration, you are my support, and you are my reason."

I honor my family and the love they have always shown me while I've been on what seems like a perpetual search for self, purpose, and a soul-throbbing quest for making a difference. The brilliant thoughts and ideas have been endless, yet they let me be me. Especially to my husband, my soul mate, my gift, it has not always been the easiest thing to do, but you have been right there by my side. I thank you for giving me the space, permission, and encouragement to "do me." I owe so much of my pursuit of life to my children. I have no doubt my life changed for the better the moment I met each of you. I could not imagine my existence without you. Your encouragement over the years has done more than you could imagine. I'm so proud to be your mom. I can hardly wait to see how you will change the world. To my parents, I am who I am because you are who you are. Your belief in me makes what I do possible. Though I am grown, you still look out for me. I'm sure I'll do the same for my trio too. My sisters and my brother are the best siblings for me. We've always done whatever it took to do whatever had to be done. Your support, handholding, laughs, and soul food cannot be measured. I've learned so much by watching and listening to you. Family has always been so important to me, and I have a big one too. I'm grateful for my entire family and the love and legacy that will always endure. I can't begin to thank you all individually but just know you are all near and dear to my heart. To my friends, girls, tribe, No Limit, and my no-matter-what accountability partner— you know who you are. I could not possibly imagine doing this life without you. We have cried in the midnight hour together, prayed the house down together, laughed until we nearly passed out, and even threatened to cut a few people and go to jail like real ride-or-die friends should. I'm more than blessed to know you. God truly hooked me up, I must have stood in the friends line twice.

To all of my coaches, each and every one of you has pushed me to be more authentic and confident, elevate my mindset, and live big. Thank you Dr. Draion Burch, the visionary leader of the Medical Mogul Academy and the class of 2020, you are truly one of a kind. To my spiritual guide, founder of the Abundant Life Path and The Coach Consortium, Rebecca Lynn Pope, affectionately referred to as my "Coaching Coach," words aren't enough to express my gratitude. Thank you for seeing in the spirit and leading me until I could see for myself. I think of you every time I buy red lipstick (wink). Blessings and abundance! To Felicia Phillips, you're one powerhouse of *a woman and truly an inspiration. I always remember your words, "It's about relationships." And it is. To Tamara Hartley, my very first coach over a decade ago, it was an experience that has since led me to thousands of hours and dozens of coaching models.*

To those who will read this book, I wrote it specifically for you. I heard you in the exam room, the hospital halls, the church pews, the conference seats, the office, the store, the car, and every other place humanity resides. I heard you, and each time, I saw a little piece of me. So, this book is dedicated to us, the ones who know we are created for greatness. We matter, we can make a difference, and we are in this quest to shine our light together. This book is about thriving from exactly where you are to where you are called to be next. There's nothing more salient than now. To everyone carrying extra weight, mentally and physically, this book is dedicated to you.

Only God knows what it took to carry, labor, and deliver this baby. I thank God, the Holy Spirit, the Universe, and all its angels for the transformations and fulfillment of this book's purpose.

Contents

Acknowledgments

This book would not have been possible and done in excellence without my reasons for writing it in the first place. All of my patients, followers, friends, family, and everyone who fueled my passion for spreading a message of health and healing made this all possible.

A sincere thanks and shout out to my One Life Support team who lived up to their name; truly, Kandace and Jean were my creative lifesavers. My publishing team, Publish Your Gift, kept this project moving forward with excellence.

Foreword

It only takes about 90 seconds with Dr. Jada to be enveloped by her light. So, whenever I introduce someone else to Dr. Jada, they all report back to me that they experienced the same feeling. Allow me to share the story of how we first met.

When I moved to Atlanta, I was eager to immerse myself in the health and wellness community of Atlanta. With this goal in mind, whenever I connected with anyone in the health field, from physicians to personal trainers to consumers of health and wellness products, I was encouraged to reach out to Dr. Jada Moore. Her name came up so many times, I knew I had to find her. I searched for her, sent emails and Facebook messages, and reached out to her assistant, with no success.

After several months of being unable to reach Dr. Jada, I received a LinkedIn connection request. It was from Dr. Jada Moore-Ruffin. I was shocked! Did she know I had been looking for her for months? I sent her a message that simply stated, "I have been looking for you." Her response was, "Well, here I am." We exchanged phone numbers, and I scheduled a time to speak with her. I told her briefly, for the sake of not wanting to sound like a stalker during our first virtual meeting, I had been trying to find her since I moved to Atlanta without success. After I told her more about myself, she asked, "Well what can I do for you?" I simply asked,

"Can I just hang around you?" She said sure. We scheduled a day to have lunch. And since that time, I haven't let go.

To say that my search for Dr. Jada was worth it is an understatement. Simply put, she is one of the most magical women I've ever met. God's hand is all over her and everything she touches. So, even though I didn't know it at the time, asking if I could just hang around her was the best and most impactful thing I could've asked for. Dr. Jada has shown me what the anointing looks like in the flesh and in the most practical sense. That anointing oozes out of her, and when she steps into a room, you can feel it. And while she recognizes her gift, she does not squander it or take it for granted but handles it with grace and responsibility.

Dr. Jada Moore-Ruffin is a board-certified family medicine physician and certified obesity medicine specialist. She has worked and served patients in a variety of clinical settings in her twenty-plus years of practicing medicine. While there are many medical professionals who assist their patients with weight loss, the reason why Dr. Jada's patients experience such great success is because of the deeper work she does with them. There are so many things in our lives that "weigh us down": an unfulfilling career, an unsatisfying relationship, stress, anxiety, a lack of purpose, and the list goes on. Dr. Jada assists her clients in unlocking and releasing these things. This, as she describes it, is the "real work." The work requires you to be honest and vulnerable, but with Dr. Jada as your guide, you are always supported. As she always says, "The physical weight loss, that's the easy part."

I am excited about Dr. Jada Moore-Ruffin's debut book, *Girl, Get Ready to Lose the Damn Weight!*, because it's an opportunity for you to experience her in that anointing, without having to search for her for months! I often tell Dr. Jada, "You're good for deep conversation, inspiration, and a good laugh!" This book gives you all those elements! No matter where you are in your health and wellness journey, this book is full of content that will take you further. This work has truly been a labor of love, and I've watched her put her entire heart into it. I'm so excited because I know for so many, your breakthrough is just on the other side of one of her chapters. Congratulations, Dr. Jada Moore-Ruffin, for seeing this all the way through! I'm so unbelievably proud of you. I am so thankful that God allowed me to find you at just the right time. I'm never letting go.

Lauren W. Powell, MD
The Culinary Doctor®

Preface

This is not your average weight loss book. It is not about the latest diet tricks. It is not about how to lose twenty pounds in twenty minutes or less. This is not a book about physical fitness, and you won't find the secret to a foolproof way to get killer abs or beautiful butts. This is not about how to look like a million bucks for a few dollars a day. Now, there's nothing wrong with those books. This is just not one of them.

Who this book is not for:

1. those who are looking for a quick fix
2. those looking to add another failure to their never-ending search for the magic potion for losing weight, again
3. those who just want to lose weight for a wedding, reunion, or photo shoot
4. those who are "perfectly fine" except for the weight
5. those who are simply not ready to take on a bigger life not just a smaller body.

Who this book is for:

1. those ready for positive change in every aspect of how you do life

2. those who want to lose the baggage that has weighed you down in life

3. those who want to discover how emotional eating feeds your weight struggle

4. those ready to confront the real problems with your weight struggle

5. those ready to go deeper, farther, and faster toward a life of peace, joy, and self-love

6. those really ready to lose ALL the weight once and for all!

This book will change your life as you engage it and use it as I guide you toward mental fitness, unemotional eating, self-support, tough love, and the reward of physical weight loss.

Prologue

This book almost didn't happen. I had planned a weekend writing retreat in a hotel on the other side of the city. All week long, I was in the zone. My energy was great! I had been sleeping, eating, exercising, getting things off my list, and preparing for the most productive weekend. I was actually excited that I would finally get my book done. I boasted God-inspired clarity and focus that was so encouraging.

I had been putting off my book writing for months. Others in my coaching cohort had finished their books or were picking out their covers, and some had even done elaborate book launches. I admired them and was inspired by them, but in a secret place within my subconscious, I felt left behind. Well, not left behind. Even worse, I felt responsible for being behind the rest of them. I had created the time gap, or so I felt. But my time had come to ink my book and jump on track.

The day I was set to start the book-writing weekend, I had a half-day in the office, one that was lighter than usual. I had an appointment with my doctor that went great. Then, later I had a meeting with my new financial advisor for our first in-person consultation. We were acquaintances of sorts, introduced by a mutual connection. Our meeting was also overdue, but that day we would get started and move things right along. Logistically speaking, this meeting was rightly placed, and I would be off to the hotel, a short drive away.

The meeting started out with the usual exchange of cordials. "Thank God it's Friday" and "How's the family?" and "Lots of rain lately." We began to get into the overview of financials. He jotted notes about business history, credit, loans, equipment, assets, expenses, etc. I felt pretty good that despite not being a number or incredibly detail-oriented person, I had most answers in my brain's immense data bank. As the meeting went on and the questions got more personal, I felt more vulnerable and the urge to self-protect from judgment. Nothing changed about the line of questioning, yet I felt myself shrinking in my seat. At a point near the close of the hour-long meeting, I began to experience a familiar yet unwanted set of feelings both physically and emotionally. My words became softer, my eyes shifted downward, my chin tilted lower, and a cold wave caused my insides to shiver. I could feel the little girl in me begin to take over my once bold presence. I wasn't proud of the numbers as he began to ask me about my income. I heard a whisper in my ear that penetrated my psyche like a bullet: "Not good enough." I was triggered. Mentally it was over for me. The meeting ended shortly thereafter, and as I walked to the parking lot, tears welled up in my eyes. The flurry of emotions began to shower me with sadness, frustration, and anger. Not only because of what felt like a financial assault but because it happened just moments before what I had planned to be one of the most celebrated times of my life.

Needless to say, the book happened. Despite setbacks, delays, missed deadlines, and all kinds of distractions, the book was born just a little after its due date. Nonetheless, in full trust of the universe and divine timing, now is the time.

Introduction

Not struggling with your weight? Well, someone close to you is. So, read this for them. Stand in the gap and use this book as a tool to understand, enlighten, encourage, love, and support those around you. Be a change agent for those around you. Obesity is the largest and most serious epidemic of our time. It's going to take a collective community to reverse the widespread devastation that obesity has created and will have on future generations.

As I was writing this book, I kept saying to myself, "Are you sure this is a book about weight loss?" And I kept replying back to myself, "Yes, of sorts." It came to me that everyone has their place in the process. I realized that my place in this book was not to go on a crusade to attack the fast food industry or lobby to have the USDA make better food laws or insist that there be reform in the public assistance programs. Now, I do have very clear views on each of those and continue to support the work being done on those platforms. However, I wanted to create a higher level of consciousness in humanity regarding how we care for ourselves and those around us. So, again, I say this is not a quick weight loss book although I have helped thousands of people implement those very weight loss strategies successfully. In fact, in my weight loss and wellness center, I continue to help people shed the physical weight, which in part inspired this book. After thousands of pounds lost, my goal is to make sure your entire life is set up to not only maintain but sustain the weight loss and enjoy a happy and fulfilling life.

Come with me as we learn how to think thinner and live lighter.

Mind

1

Those Damn Triggers

A trigger ignites like a match to a flame.

A trigger is like someone pouring salt on an open wound. It causes an immediate surge of pain. The action could be a word, sound, smell, taste, or color; it could be anything in any shape, form, or fashion that resonates with your senses. The reaction is almost immediate, intense, intrusive, and often persistent. See, the problem with triggers is that they are a function of memory that keeps showing up in the present. The Urban Dictionary (which I actually happen to like) defines a trigger as "a term used to describe sensations, images, or experiences that cause a traumatic memory." Triggers keep us connected to our unwanted and often repressed past.

A while back, somewhere probably in childhood or even infancy, something happened, and you didn't like it. You created a story or an associated way of dealing with the situation. You stored this away in your brain's permanent data bank. That became your default way of recognizing and handling that feeling whenever it came up again. It was not taught; it was learned.

I'm reminded of a story shared by one of my patients who was a survivor of sexual assault in her early twenties while working as an extern in China. At the time, she was living her best life, exploring the world and making a difference in the creative and artistic world of movement and dance. One night she was hanging out with other US locals. After a few drinks, she caught a ride home with a guy she knew from other hangouts. Instead of taking her back to her quaint bungalow on the outskirts of the city, he took her to a dark alley hidden away from the mainstream hustle and bustle. She recalled the smell of the sushi on his fingertips as he held his hand over her mouth. She could feel the warmth of the summer air mixed with the moist heat from his body pressed against her. She could see the half-moon staring down at her helpless frame yet refusing to come to her rescue. A wave of chill bumps lined her perfectly shaped arms as she boarded the plane for a long flight home. Her soul felt empty and void, mourning the loss of normalcy she left behind on foreign soil. She survived, but the vibrant, innocent, and free-spirited girl she once knew did not. Her life today at forty is great some days, horrible some days, and "just is" on some days. To this day, the slightest aroma of sushi makes her sick to her stomach. Most summer days are fine, but occasionally when the night air is just so, her soul registers that exact temperature and humidity like the night that changed her life forever. She stays home on those nights, reaching for whatever will comfort her through the moment.

Triggers can even happen when you least expect them to, on a stage, in a movie, at the most inconvenient times.

As we get older, they don't seem to have the same sting they once did, but they are still there. They have an aftereffect, causing us to walk through life cautiously to avoid them. Some of us find ways around them, ignore them, suppress them, or react to them.

No matter what, in the moment, they stand to rob us of our power and steal our joy. In many cases, we just hand over our joy.

Going forward, look for your triggers. Resist the urge to avoid, ignore, suppress, or react to them. Become familiar with them. Learn how to spot them on command. Embrace them and then give them purpose. Speak to them, create a simple phrase like this. "I recognize you for what you were for me. I no longer need your reminders of my past. Now, I have other work to do, and your new purpose is to help me out. You can do that by giving me a reason to help others who've experienced this."

Girl, Get Ready! Lesson #1:

Don't curse your triggers; bless them then redefine them.

Action Step #1:

Sometimes, there may be a direct correlation like the patient I mentioned. Sometimes, there is an indirect association with the feeling although the trigger may not represent a specific moment in your past. Use my example of being triggered during my financial advisor meeting. I was triggered by words. I felt like I wasn't good enough.

By now, you may recall an experience that left you with unpleasant memories. If it's ever shown up again, when was it, where were you, what did you notice about your face, body sensations, and thoughts?

2

Trash Negative Thinking

Drop the loser mentality! You are the captain of your life and MVP of your own team; lead yourself like a winner.

Does anyone come to mind when someone says, "She's a Negative Nancy?" Maybe you have been on a work team and whenever a new idea is tossed out, you can count on this one person to shoot it down before it even hits the table. Perhaps, when you see an incoming call from a friend, your first instinct is to let it go to voicemail because you just know you'll get the daily rundown on all that's wrong with the world today. I know I certainly have. According to the *Oxford Dictionary*, the word "negative" means "to characterize something by the absence of rather than the presence of its distinguishing characteristics, to refuse, reject, or veto." Just saying the word "negative" aloud causes a sense of heaviness and dread.

If something is not going our way, a lot of times, we are filtering this experience as either bad or not good. In a split second, before we even recognize it, we've issued a judgment on each thing that comes our way. The brain quickly processes and summarizes in a way that translates something as lacking potential, promise, or purpose. These are the three Ps of negative thinking. When does it happen? It happens when we process the world around us as bad, wrong, and limited.

Negative thinking can almost become a way of life. If we don't see the potential, promise, or purpose, then we just say no or turn our minds off when we see things that way. The thinking then connects to a reciprocal feeling, thereby causing us to respond with emotions of despair and lack. So, in essence, we continue to attract more of the same. It doesn't get any better either because we get caught in what I call "Negative Loops" that keep going round and round without an exit door.

People who operate like this seldom see it in themselves. That's the hard part. All too often, negative-minded people can slip into the victim mode really quickly. And victim mode is a hallmark sign of underlying negative thought patterns. This is in fact its own category of negative thinking—it's the victim mentality. This form is somewhat deceiving too because the words that come out or even the actions of "the victim" may not always jump out at you. This person actually believes in themselves but not in others. There's the impression that when bad things happen, someone else is to blame. They have lost the ability to take responsibility for outcomes, often rendering themselves powerless because the power belongs to the perpetrator who caused the effect. When you lose the ability to be a cause in the effects of your life, then there's limited room to create what you want. So, if we go back to the three Ps of negative thinking and whether it's you or someone you come into contact with, negative thoughts are contagious and sickening—think viral. And trust me, no matter how positive and happy-go-lucky you claim to be, we've all been guilty of it. Let me prove it to you!

Girl, Get Ready! Lesson #2:

Check your thoughts and trash negative words; replace them with "yes, can, and possible" statements.

Action Step #2:

Let's do a self-check. Take three sticky notes and on each square write down one thing that causes you to feel despair or lack. Don't complicate this exercise. Is it a failing relationship? Struggles with your weight? Working on a job you hate? Living paycheck to paycheck? Whatever it is, quickly jot them down. Now, look at the first one, then close your eyes and think about the word on the sticky note. What thoughts begin to surface? Ah ha, told you!

Begin to understand negative thinking by seeing these key-words come up in your thoughts or conversations. Wrong, bad, broke, hate, fat, and even simple nondescript words like no, nobody, not, neither, can't, never, none, and nothing can infect your vocabulary whether verbally or nonverbally. The more you use them, the more likely it is that you could be the one being sent straight to voicemail. Check yourself often. Ask your honest friend (we all should have at least one) to do the sticky notes for you if you can't.

3

Surviving Self-Sabotage

Stop being the victim in your own narrative.

Let's break this down. Imagine this scenario. You're in the car rushing to a meeting, and it looks like the angels are on your side. You're actually making good time, hitting all the green lights, and by some act of God, the traffic is moving at a nice steady pace. You get off at the exit, and you're approaching the final turn to your destination, and then the arms to the railroad crossing safety gate are lowered just over the hood of your car. You realize everything that previously worked out for you to make your meeting on time was just canceled out when the rail arms were lowered. I know I've had that feeling, like something out there just won't let me be great.

Now, let's apply that analogy to a different scenario. Tonya, one of my weight loss clients, was known for having a great run at following the custom weight loss plan we had created for her. She would reach her weekly goal, we'd talk about her success, and a few weeks later she would hit a wall, and I'd notice a plateau in both her weight and her motivation. Then she'd pick up again, and then she'd plateau again. After tracking this for a couple of months, in our next coaching session, I brought to Tonya's attention that I had noticed this trend in her results. At first, she was dismissive about the observation and blew it off as just a coincidence. I continued to push Tonya, a corporate executive, to explore more about what may be getting in the way of her consistent success. Finally, she broke down in tears and shared that she was so excited about her progress and when others would notice, she would become afraid that she would not be able to maintain the results once she reached her goal. So, she would find herself reverting back to old habits whenever this would come up for her.

In other words, getting back to the first analogy, she was moving right along, hitting all the green lights, coasting on the highway, and then the safety guard rails would lower just as she was approaching the last turn into the parking lot. This time, it wasn't the random occurrence of railway sensors coming down to protect Tonya from the oncoming train. It was Tonya, putting up unintentional protective behaviors as obstacles to keep her from feeling the sense of short-lived success she was programming her mind to create. She was successful in most areas of her life but had not been able to conquer her weight for fear of success and then failure. All along, I suspected this was the case. I had seen it all too often, especially in my clients who are high achievers. I coached her through these self-imposed obstacles called self-sabotage, and she began to see consistent results that she could eventually embrace and build in her goals for physical wellness.

Self-sabotaging behaviors have many origins. It commonly happens to high achievers and people with perfectionist tendencies, whether you see yourself as such or not. Whenever we sense a threat, we go into defense mode. In this case, we'd rather set ourselves up than let others see our shortcomings, vulnerabilities, and failures.

Girl, Get Ready! Lesson #3:

Don't be careful in one area of your life and careless in another.

Action Step #3:

Explore your self-sabotaging behaviors. Where have you made it a habit to defend yourself, from yourself, by attacking yourself first?

4

Harnessing Unforgiveness

*Let it go so you can move ahead with
what you really want.*

We've heard before that the love of money is the root of all evil. I believe the lack of forgiveness is the root of all suffering. When I first began to explore areas of unforgiveness in my life, I was at a weekend coaching retreat I had enrolled in several weeks prior while at an open house that one of my doctor friends had invited me to. We weren't incredibly close but had shared some intimate conversations about our upbringing and unresolved personal issues. At the time, I had this incredibly busy life: I'm a wife and a mom of three kids, and I had just started my own business. The last thing I had time to do was spend an entire weekend in a group coaching retreat. But she insisted I try it! Knowing that I was in a new season in my career, I figured maybe it could help me be a better entrepreneur—and besides, there were hundreds of people registered for the course. I concluded, if nothing else, I could manage to pass out a few business cards and maybe pick up a few new clients.

At the retreat, several people were summoned to the microphone to "share." One guy in the room shared a point, and the course leader countered with a point that I thought watered down the previous point. So, I simply raised my hand in support of my unknown classmate, and the next thing I know, I was summoned to the front of the room with 226 faces staring at me awaiting my "share," which I had no intentions of sharing. The course leader asked me a couple of questions, and before I knew it, I was sobbing at the microphone, sharing about an incident in my childhood that apparently resulted in some unforgiveness that had shown up in various ways throughout my wildly successful adult life. I had not tapped into this fallacy and in fact considered myself to have at the very least a decent relationship with my parents.

During the retreat, I learned so much about how unforgiveness had taken root in my life and at times had undermined my emotional well-being. In all my work and experiences in facilitating the healing of others through the years, unforgiveness had often been found as the source of persistent suffering, pain, and distress in so many ways, showing up as binge eating, poor spending habits, fragile relationships, divorce, and distant parenting, to name a few.

In some cases, mental images of a perpetrator may immediately pop up, especially if that memory is so heavily embedded in the present reality that not a day goes by that one isn't reminded of the circumstances that led to lingering feelings of bitterness. However, in so many people, the wounds are so deeply embedded, or experiences are so profoundly repressed, that forgiveness doesn't even seem necessary.

Believe it or not, often the person we need to forgive is ourselves. When working with patients, clients, and even myself, I've discovered we have ongoing areas of remorse and discontent because of things we have done or things we may not have done, for that matter. In one case, I worked with a client who got pregnant in college, which she chose to terminate by having an abortion without ever telling her family. She moved on from that juvenile relationship, completed college, and married the man of her dreams, only to later struggle with infertility. She was never able to become pregnant again. Despite being an accomplished executive, financially established, and socially active, she could not reason with her guilt that had now become laced with feelings of inadequacy.

For over a decade, struggles with her weight would become her biggest symptom of a life lived with unforgiveness. The number on the scale would go up and down like an elevator, especially when her marriage was buckling under the unacknowledged pressure of not being able to conceive. After trials of in vitro fertilization, hormone shots, and dozens of pregnancy tests, she was exasperated, emotionally fragile, and notably overweight. Whether shortcomings were real or perceived, she could not get over the malady of barrenness.

She eventually found herself on the doorsteps of a therapist's office, and after months of sobbing and leaving the therapist's office feeling like she only relived her pain with each visit, she came into my office for a weight loss consultation. The moment I saw her, even at an arm's length, separated by a dark wooden desk, I could sense the mental exhaustion and see the physical repository of her pain. I just knew she would need more than a weight loss plan. After the consultation, I recommended an intense hybrid coaching program that would focus just as much on her healing as it would on her health. She agreed. Shortly into our coaching, the truth began to unravel, and we began to keenly focus on what would be a key to unlocking the door to success—forgiveness.

Once we began to do the work, she began to see how unforgiveness had trapped her into a way of seeing herself as a failure no matter how much she achieved. She acknowledged never feeling as though she deserved to become pregnant because of the abortion and had accepted infertility as God's way of punishing her for the past abomination. We spent several weeks coaching her through those self-crucifying beliefs, chartering a path to forgiveness, and opening channels of self-love. She eventually lost sixty-four pounds, got remarried, and adopted a beautiful baby girl who she and her husband took straight home from the newborn nursery.

Kendala's story reminds us of this: Not until we intentionally open the doors on the closets that hide our skeletons, excavate the graves where our secrets have been buried, and confront the situations that have caused us pain are we able to find the path to true peace.

Girl, Get Ready! Lesson #4:

Unforgiveness is the root of all suffering.

Action Step #4:

Search and find 10 ways unforgiveness may show up in your everyday life.

Find (Un)forgiveness

S	B	M	T	L	I	U	G	P	R	O	A	U	S
P	E	L	E	I	O	T	N	H	S	E	S	P	N
I	S	S	A	I	H	S	M	R	S	M	H	S	R
H	D	B	I	M	E	A	F	O	E	A	A	R	N
S	L	I	E	M	E	Y	D	N	N	R	M	S	H
N	N	U	O	E	P	N	D	S	D	N	E	L	R
O	R	T	E	T	R	M	L	A	A	H	L	R	M
I	R	M	I	S	U	M	S	A	S	U	I	R	E
T	A	P	L	S	T	F	R	I	R	R	E	R	B
A	M	T	S	I	L	N	T	O	U	T	O	E	A
L	F	R	U	S	T	R	A	T	I	O	N	A	E
E	R	R	S	D	M	S	W	O	R	R	Y	R	M
R	R	E	S	E	N	T	M	E	N	T	H	T	R
S	T	I	R	I	R	R	L	O	A	T	N	T	L

SADNESS
BLAME
WORRY
FRUSTRATION
RELATIONSHIPS
HURT
GUILT
RESENTMENT
SHAME

For more information, go to www.girlgetreadybook.com

5

Recognizing Boredom

If you are bored with your life, do something about it.

Boredom is what I call the "camouflage emotion." Yes, boredom is an emotion, and it often is wrapped in discontentment. This is true across the lifespan, and in fact, boredom is one of the telltale signs of adolescent depression. It can be found in children who experience attention disorders. It hides out in adults who job hop, overeat, and constantly complain.

Being bored translates to being unhappy and will almost always have a root cause. It has an insidious nature; in other words, it comes about in a gradual, subtle way but almost always is associated with harmful effects. And true to form, you can count on these harmful effects to be elusive as well. What does that mean? It means a person could go months, years, even decades with seemingly insignificant movement in life because there's a lack of interest in your life as it is. There follows complacency, which has a ripple effect for not only you but for everyone connected to you.

Working with clients through the years, I have identified three types of boredom:

1. **Classic Boredom**: The classically bored person will tend to daydream, drift off, and manage a very routine

existence. There is a low level of creativity and a tendency to hide behind the thoughts of complacency and contentment. A classically bored person will rarely challenge themselves to reach for a higher standard.

2. **Frenetic Boredom**: This is almost paradoxical in description. It's like busy boredom. In these cases, there's a tendency to be antsy, often looking for something to do. There's a persistent nag at play that is hard to ignore, so when left unaddressed, the mind begins to wander, looking for something to do. I often find this behavior in people I describe as "grazers."

3. **Apathetic Boredom**: This can sometimes be mistaken for or be a tip off of underlying depression or depressive features. A telltale sign is the commonly used phrase, "I don't care." This hallmark is lack of interest, lack of enthusiasm, and lack of concern for work, play, and other activities or tasks of daily functioning. This is common in teens and will often spill over into I-don't-care attitudes about health, body image, or hygiene. There's such a penetrating level of disengagement that the behavior takes on a "checked-out" demeanor.

Why is boredom so pervasive? It's because it's easier to stick with the status quo and not move forward. We have become conditioned to choose easy over hard. What does this have to do with weight loss? It's simple. Being bored may translate to dissatisfaction, and without dealing with the root of the emotion, eating fills a void and delivers immediate satisfaction.

The two ways I often recommend addressing boredom are 1) building mental fitness and 2) tapping into the physical connection. Start by observing your actions to create awareness. Some keywords to look for in your thoughts, conversations, and actions include: don't care, routine, sameness, unconcern, apathy, weariness, dullness, restlessness, monotony, indifference, lethargy.

Fatigue and low energy are sure to follow the classically bored person. Begin to shift this pattern by adding or adjusting physical activity to increase energy. It doesn't have to be marathon running or kickboxing. You may not have that physical ability or an interest in those high-intensity activities, and that's fine. Just get into something and do it daily. Group classes like Zumba, aerobics, or cycling are good options to improve both physical and mental boredom. Having to learn new routines, interact with people, and change accountability are good incentives for the classically bored. Those with frenetic boredom can benefit from yoga, Pilates, or high-intensity interval training (HIIT) activities that offer a change of routine, like a daily workout with different activities each day. This way, there's enough variety and intrigue to keep your interest piqued and motivation high. To overcome apathetic boredom, strengthen your mental and physical core with activities like yoga, Pilates, golf, rowing, or tennis.

We give up a little part of our destiny each day. A teeny, tiny piece of our big work on Earth fades away, not as a function of time but as a function of effect. If you're holding back on something you're supposed to be doing, creating, or being, then you are causing a hold-up for someone else connected to you. Maybe that's your kids, your husband, your cubicle mate, or your neighbor, but I submit to you that your impact is even greater and goes beyond the people you know to people you don't even know.

Girl, Get Ready! Lesson #5:

Boredom is not innocent; it can lead to a trail of destruction.

Action Step #5:

Examine your patterns. Do you find comfort in food? Which of the patterns described in this chapter have you experienced in the past? Write them down.

6

Losing Limiting Beliefs

*The only reason you can't is because
you don't believe you can.*

Have you ever had an idea or situation come up and the first thing that comes to mind is "That will never work" or "That's an awful idea" or "I don't have enough…" or "I tried that once and…"? I know I have. I've thought or said those very words over a thousand times. If you look really carefully, I'm willing to bet that you have also uttered these thoughts or words at some point in your life. These constructs rise out of the endless fountain of what are called limiting beliefs. What is a limiting belief? It is an inherent convention in your mental makeup that sees but only so far before it stops. A limiting belief is a capacity issue. It's like an empty and full mark on your gas hand. The tank can only go so low or the car will turn off. On the other hand, the gas tank can only contain so much before the gas pump hits its full capacity, then spills over and shuts off.

We have often been taught that there's a low mark and a high mark to just about anything. We've been trained to avoid falling too low. Whatever you do, don't come in last place. I recall a little running joke in our family from when my boys were running track a number of years ago. They may not appreciate this story, so unless they read the book, this is our little secret. My oldest was about ten years old, and his coach had decided to try him at the 400-meter race, which was a bit long for his liking. He practiced for hours during the week. He and one other teammate ran the same race, so they practiced together and ran side by side during the track competitions. It became commonplace for the two boys to have their own race almost as if there were no other boys competing in the race. From the stands, it looked as though they were both battling for next to last place, as if they had fixed in their minds, "I can't be the last." They expected that the coach would be upset, and of course, nobody wants to be last. But I wonder if they ever considered that, in fact, they were both actually in competition for first place!

By the same token, we've been conditioned to not reach too high, for "too high" is the place where failure hangs out. That's where disappointment is lurking around. Too high is a trap, and it should only be tested by the foolish. That's the all or none zone, the eat or be eaten world, or in some cases, we make aiming too high as costly as life or death in our minds.

I have at times found myself in this very same dilemma. Whenever I have taken on what I call "living big," I would have those sometimes fleeting and at other times lingering thoughts of "Can I really pull this off?" I immediately begin counting the cost of the what ifs. When I started my business, I was a struggling solopreneur who stepped out on a wing and a prayer to break loose from the traditional model of the healthcare system. Growth was slow but steady. If you've been in the entrepreneur's seat for any period of time, you can imagine exactly what this feels like. Having left a six-figure job as a medical director for a community health center, I was literally starting over at the bottom.

I had a business coach, a couple of them in fact, and would regularly meet for progress updates and new strategy planning. In one of our meetings, my coach could sense the despair and corresponding exhaustion from the tone in my voice. Typically, I am the high-energy optimist, and my demeanor that day was way off center. She asked me a few questions and gave a few pointers, yet I had not completely turned my attitude around. Next she asked, "What do you think is the problem?" I replied, "Instead of playing to win, I'm playing not to lose." I had no idea that was my position until that moment. I learned from that day forward that those two scenarios are not one and the same. Playing to win is very, very different from playing not to lose. In essence, I was contending for next to last place. I had not given myself permission, regardless of the bottom line or what I had or didn't have, to compete for first place. I was spending the same amount of time and energy, if not more, to battle not to lose or fail as it would take to fight my way to the front of the race.

In October 2002, the New York Jets' head coach, Herman Edwards, sat in his usual weekly press conference with the media, this time at the helm of a team smack dab in the middle of a losing season. The well-regarded football coach was asked cordially by a reporter if he would have to talk to his team about giving up on the season. And Edwards's passionate rebuttal would make a permanent mark in history. Known for his successful years as a player and then as a coach, he went into a resounding statement about quitting summarized by the poignant quote that has been stated time and time again in the world of sports and borrowed in many mantles of leadership, "YOU PLAY TO WIN THE GAME!"

Most of us will shoot for the middle, the safe space, the norm, the place where everyone else can be found. Every single time we have a "too high" thought, the Mindset Safety Patrol whispers into our ears, "Now, wait a second. Don't you think that's a little dangerous?" And we reply at lightning speed, "Yes, I do! I'd better back off. This could go bad. I'm out of my league. I have to stay in the safe zone."

The only reason these concepts exist is because we have put limits on our capacity. Somewhere along the way, we place an empty and a full mark on our potential. And that is what we use to monitor or patrol our limits from any place and in any way. Of all the personal obstacles I see in the way of people's quest toward better health, weight loss, joyful relationships, purposeful careers, and abundant living, the most resilient intruder is limiting beliefs.

Girl, Get Ready! Lesson #6:

Lose limiting beliefs, so you can win at the game of life.

Action Step #6:

Say this prayer:

God, because you are the master crafter and I am your masterpiece, I know I am created for greatness. Remove every limitation I have put on myself and those I have allowed others to put on my potential. Help me to burst through the invisible seal of my capacity. Let me see in myself what you see in me.

7

Ditching Procrastination

*Nobody ever won a marathon sitting down
thinking about running.*

I once read a poem, and it went something like this:

> *If you had started a year ago,*
>
> *You would be a year ahead.*
>
> *If you had started six months ago,*
>
> *You would be six months ahead.*
>
> *If you had started three months ago,*
>
> *You would be three months ahead,*
>
> *But you didn't.*
>
> *Instead you did nothing,*
>
> *And so, nothing changed*
>
> *And it never will . . .*
>
> ~ Unknown ~

Raise your hand if you know ANYONE who struggles with procrastination. This is a big one when it comes to thinking thinner and living lighter. I've learned over the years that procrastination can rob you of your peace, steal your confidence, squander opportunity, and waste your precious time.

Those four in combination can ruin your life if you let it get out of hand. The nature of procrastination is that it gives this false sense of security that later not only exists but is also better than the immediate present. Now, let's be clear; we're not talking about careful contemplation about a life-altering decision or action. We're talking about the sum of many little things that go undone because we put them off. I really want you to get this because if you're fortunate enough to be a procrastinator, you have some really unique qualities that you may have overlooked that could move you toward recovery.

I use the term "recovering procrastinator" because procrastination for many is a default plan, and for that reason alone, we have to work at "unprocrastination," the opposite of which is action not reaction. Often procrastinators are waiting for a consequence—in other words, a reason or catalyst to act. So we must first feel the impact *before* we address the issue. An oversimplification is that we must feel the heat of the fire before we install the smoke detector. Procrastination is made up of a simple yet complex trap. For more information, go to www.girlgetreadybook.com.

Often, when I do one-on-one weight loss consultations with prospective clients, we discover their weight problems started years ago. In one case, Kendra had experienced a thirty-pound weight gain after starting a new job at a major university four years prior. She had done well in her new role but found it to be increasingly more demanding over the previous six months. She had stopped weighing herself on the scale because it was just too depressing to watch the numbers creep up. When Kendra finally came into my office, she had gained an additional 17 pounds and was weighing in at 247 pounds. She had been recently diagnosed with pre-diabetes, formerly called borderline diabetes, a condition in which the body doesn't metabolize glucose (blood sugar) effectively, which results in excess glucose in the bloodstream or diabetes. She knew she had a family history of diabetes from both of her parents yet had not really considered she would develop it. After all, she was in her forties, and other than feeling tired all the time, she felt fine. Now, she was facing diabetes and a body mass index (BMI) that put her in the Extreme Obesity category.

In hindsight, Kendra acknowledged that she had been really busy at work, kept putting off getting her regular checkups, and ignored her body's signs of distress. She admitted that she had reluctantly bought larger clothes each year for the past three years because she could no longer fit anything in her closet. She was frustrated every time she had to get dressed for a presentation. She felt like others were looking at her, secretly talking about her size, and she even believed she had been overlooked for major projects to advance her career because of her weight.

I congratulated Kendra for taking these first steps to take control of her health. Then I confidently reassured Kendra that she was in the right place, and I was certain we could help her set and achieve her goals. Together we developed a wellness plan for her, and she started the journey to lose the weight, improve her health, restore her confidence, and enjoy success in every aspect of her life.

Let's walk through Kendra's Procrastination Trap. For a more detailed description, go to www.girlgetreadybook.com.

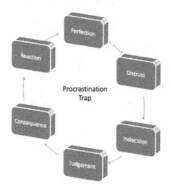

Perfection: Kendra was waiting for the perfect time to take off work to get a checkup.

Indecision: Kendra knew she was gaining weight but couldn't decide what to do about it.

Distrust: Kendra began to lose trust in the scale because it would often reveal to her what she didn't want to see, so she stopped using it.

Judgment: Kendra felt badly about and lost confidence in herself, and she often felt others judged her too.

Consequence: Kendra experienced prediabetes, fatigue, low self-confidence, additional clothing expenses, and a lack of job and career progress.

Reaction: Kendra was frustrated about taking new medications, making forced decisions, and feeling a lack of control.

Girl, Get Ready! Lesson #7:

Procrastination is the thief of success.

Action Step #7:

Write out a procrastination formula using your own life. Identify one area in which you have put off doing something important using the example above.

8

Break Up with Busyness

Busy is fake news.

Busyness is now America's biggest pastime. Not to be mistaken with "business," as in occupation or ownership in an enterprise, "busyness" is more like a state of being and has been described as the condition of having a great deal to do. Busyness is a byproduct of little time and lots of stuff crunched into the regulated boxes on a calendar. No matter who we are, how much money we make, how many degrees we've earned, or how many people recognize our face, we are all subjected to the same square box, and increment of time called a day. Yes, twenty-four hours are our daily allotment, nothing more and nothing less if we are so fortunate. Many of us find the need to "make the most" of every moment, or at least that's the story we tell. We intently occupy our time with work, activities, meetings, courses, and events. It would seem objectively wrong not to do so. After all, we live in the internet age, and in the flick of the wrist, we can be in any part of the world with as little as a handheld device called a smartphone. So when opportunity knocks, we can simply pick up our phones and answer.

Being busy has become a bit of a commodity. Everybody wants it. It's almost like a badge of honor. Perpetual preoccupation seems to produce receipts validating our individual value. Personally, being busy may symbolize a sense of self-worth and success. I hear it from clients and patients all the time. They are literally so busy that they don't have time to eat, work out, meditate, take a vacation, or do anything that offers any personal benefit. Then, they complain about the whole thing as if someone else has busied up their lives. I've often challenged patients by asking, if you have no time for any of the things you really either need to do or want to do, then when will you make the time?

Now, I can feel fully justified and not indignant on the matter because I've had to ask myself the same question at times. Known for "being busy," I find that people would call me on the phone and when I answer would start apologetically saying, "I know you're really busy, but . . ." At first, I would counter by saying, "Well yes, I am, but how can I help you?" Then, I began to take notice that my close friends would preface a call or text with the same phrase. My family members would too. One day I had to stop long enough to do a little self-check. If I'm seemingly too busy and they take a chance on reaching out to me, how many times have I missed connecting with them because they thought their needs were not as important as the task I was attending to and opted not to call at all? I had to really look at how that felt and how they must feel as if they are intruding on my busy life every time they simply wanted to share a funny story or let off a bit of steam. I made it a priority to reach out first. I created a list of people who I would call or text whenever I had a break in my day or on my commute. Rather than listen to the radio or jump on a business call, I committed to showing a genuine interest in what others were up to and find ways to be more thoughtful and deliberate about showing people that I wasn't too busy for them.

Getting caught up in the busy matrix can happen very easily. One major way this can sneak up on us is when we have not mastered the art of saying one short and simple word, N-O. Sometimes, that even means saying no to yourself. See, we busy people have to be careful because being constantly in motion and having a million things on our plates becomes second nature. On top of that, it can resemble somewhat of an addiction. When we're not as busy as we're accustomed to, then we begin to crave or in some respects even attract more stuff to do until we create that familiar sense of overwhelm and chaos.

A number of years ago, I attended a conference in Las Vegas with a colleague. The room was filled with doctors and other healthcare professionals who worked in community healthcare. One of the lecturers was a well-known expert in the field of psychosocial health. As he poured out from his seemingly endless fountain of knowledge, he talked extensively about findings in the research of adverse childhood events, a topic I was relatively familiar with. At a certain point in the lecture, he asked attendees to share parts of their childhood that still bore difficult emotions. Many people raised their hands, and a few shared specifics. Then he began to share some of his own personal story. He discovered in therapy that he was a workaholic, which by the way is not an actual clinical diagnosis but closely associated with clinical diagnoses in the addiction spectrum. In fact, workaholism is an addiction to work. Many of us are accustomed to having a strong work ethic and are undeniably hard workers; however, there is a distinction between working hard and work addiction. One key difference is that people who are hard workers are driven to do a good job but are not driven *by* the job. Oftentimes, work addicts will displace all other priorities like family commitments, personal well-being, vacation time, and even downtime. Even when hanging out at family events, going to children's recitals, or playing a game of golf with friends, the workaholic has their mind on work and work responsibilities, losing the ability to be present in any other setting.

Research has shown that the seeds of work addiction are often planted in childhood with children who grew up in households with an alcoholic parent or similar family dysfunctions. Those feelings of "not good enough" will also propel one into their work at a pathological pace in an effort to prove or control their perceptions of self-value.

One other common cause of excessive busyness is lack of boundaries. I'm a firm believer that you teach people how to treat you by how you treat yourself. So having very loose boundaries or no boundaries serves as an indicator to others that there are no rules of engagement and gives silent permission to create their own patterns using the trial and error method. In other words, when you are approached for requests, favors, or assignments and if you never say no but always say yes and make accommodations in order to fulfill the unwanted demands on your time, energy, or resources, you develop a template for people to follow when interacting with you. Whether the cause of busyness is related to work, not saying no, lack of boundaries, or any other reason, it can take a toll on your health, relationships, and overall sense of fulfillment and well-being.

Brain science experts estimate that the mind thinks between 60,000 to 80,000 thoughts a day. That's an average of 2,500 to 3,300 thoughts per hour. However, according to scientists, the brain can only entertain about four thoughts at once and sometimes less than that as we get older. However, other research shows that we actually are not focused on multiple things but shifting focus very rapidly, almost instantaneously. So in the era of skillful multitasking, we are actually splitting the activation of the parts of the brain, namely the prefrontal cortex that is responsible for transmitting thoughts into action and memory. This splitting happens quickly over and over in our busy minds and becomes physiologically taxing on the brain. Though we may be working on multiple tasks, this often leads to more errors, less accuracy, and accelerated fatigue, which in the end may not be as productive as we think.

If I had a dollar for every client I've seen who is up during the night with racing thoughts from the day before, the day ahead, a month from now, I'd be quite wealthy. It's never-ending. This interrupts quality sleep, and most of us aren't getting enough hours in bed in the first place. So now, we're in bed less and runaway thinking is taking over the quality of our sleep. I'm not a brain scientist, but I hypothesize that our brains are still trying to process those 80,000 thoughts caught up in a backlog!

INTERCESSION

God, help me to separate the important from the unimportant, the necessary from the unnecessary, the busy from the productive, and the yes from the no. Give me the support I need to carry out your assignments and purpose, knowing only then will I add value to my life and to the lives of those around me.

Girl, Get Ready! Lesson #8:

Honor yourself enough to say no. Saying no is an act of love and brings us closer to freedom.

Action Step #8:

Breaking up with busy behaviors can free up more time to do what you need, what you want, and what you love to do. Make a list of things you do regularly that you don't want to do. Think of a way to eliminate, reduce, or delegate those tasks.

9

Committing to Consistency

*If you have clothes of every size in your closet,
you have a consistency problem.*

Have you noticed that those bad habits you struggle to break and the things you don't want to do are the things you naturally do without a thought? When it comes to those routines and choices, it takes nothing to be consistent. Without fail, those are the things we tend to do naturally and with ease. Let's say, for example, you have committed to getting up early for morning workouts five days a week. After preparing the night before, morning comes, and you hit the snooze button four times before rolling out of bed. You know that you made a new commitment, yet your old habits got in the way and now it seems impossible to make good on hopping out of bed for workouts. However, look at another view of this scenario. You prepare the night before, and when the alarm goes off the first time, you get up immediately, get dressed, and head out to the gym, complete your workout, and go back home feeling accomplished and ready to tackle the rest of the day. This feeling of accomplishment fuels the desire to stick with the new plan.

Now, on the contrary, by holding on to the old habits of snoozing the alarm or snuggling back under the comfy blanket, you're held up by what you are experiencing in the moment, letting temporary benefit stand in the way of the long-range goals. Without lasting change, your health suffers, energy stays low, clothes don't fit well, and the sense of well-being begins to wane. This leaves you feeling unaccomplished, frustrated, and stuck with the hand you've been dealt.

Since commitment is a function of consistency, you must be able to incorporate both into your lifestyle, simultaneously and in equal parts. In other words, you can't reasonably have extraordinary commitment but lousy consistency and expect results.

I'm reminded of our new patient intake form; there is a question that asks, "How important is your goal of losing weight?" Almost always, the eager client selects ten on a scale of one to ten, from least to most important. The next question asked is, "Are you able to commit time on one day a week to meet with your Weight Loss Coach?" Alternately, a significant number of answers would be no, sometimes, or maybe. Occasionally, there would be brief explanations scribbled into the margins. Already, the commitment was wearing off.

When I was writing this book, I had spurts of enthusiasm, thoughts, and ideas, and sometimes, I would put them in my notes on my phone, or sometimes I'd just try to remember them for the next time I was able to sit down and write. At the time, I was running two businesses, working part-time for the City of Atlanta, launching my new coaching programs, and managing my family life with three kids, a husband, and a dog. If that doesn't describe a full— better yet, overflowing—plate, your superwoman cape is sturdier than mine!

I had pushed my manuscript deadline back three months already, and all I could see was another unmet deadline in my future. I felt so disappointed, frustrated, and defeated most of the time. Over a span of four months, I used a bunch of excuses: writer's block, losing and training new employees in the business, increasing demands at my other job, daylight savings time, no help keeping the kitchen clean—you name it. One night, I was making my bed while listening to one of my coaching call replays. My coach said to the group, "You've got to be consistent if you're ever going to finish your book. You've got to write even when you don't think you have anything to write." Writing is like working a muscle; the more you exercise it, the stronger you get. it. Simply put, it hit me that the same principle I teach in consistency for my weight loss patients was turned around and pointed directly at me for writing my book. I knew full well the benefits of consistency in weight loss, and over the years, I had seen my patients undergo transformations by consistently practicing the strategies my team and I taught them. I knew full well that's how I achieved my own victories over controlling my weight for the past two decades. In fact, that had been my secret sauce for achieving so many of my life's accomplishments. I had not been successful because of fleeting luck, chance, or happenstance. No, commitment and consistency lead to results. I realized I had to use this same approach to get this book done.

I had to commit to consistency. So, that's exactly what I did. I set a new deadline based on my writing schedule, not some random date I pulled out of the sky because it seemed like enough time. By having a writing schedule, I could plan to write one hour a day, averaging 500 to 750 words per hour during a good, focused writing session. By doing that seven days a week, I would have 3,500 to 5,250 words per week! In just four weeks, my book would be complete! I already had over half of it done, and with this new plan, finishing this book would be a breeze. Just knowing how I would get it done created such a sense of relief; hope proved to be the key to unlocking my writer's block.

How many of you know that these kinds of break-throughs, no matter how solid they are, can be remodeled in a matter of minutes when hit with resistance? And, you can best believe, the moment you're up to something big, there will be what I call "the smalls" marching in to bring you back down to size. So remember all of those other commitments I mentioned earlier? The businesses, job, kids, husband, and dog were all still there. My resistance was, "Exactly when can you possibly spare a whole hour each day to write?" I chuckle thinking back. The voice in my head was like that from the old school sitcom *Sanford and Son*, when Fred Sanford would look at his son, Lamont, and lead with "You big dummy" before belittling him for his bright ideas. After laughing it off, I realized the resistance to change was the problem. When I really took a closer look at my pace, I realized that I could use some serious rerouting in my routine and in my schedule across the board. For that ridiculous question, I had a simple answer. I would create a new routine to accommodate my new plan, thereby removing the resistance to change.

My plate was overflowing, in part, because I had begun to lose sight of my priorities, both personal and professional. As new things were adding to my growing list of things to do, the rate of getting things off my list was not keeping the same cadence. I was accomplishing things daily, weekly, and monthly, but it felt grueling. I needed to change how I got things done, not just how much I got done.

Already an early riser, my mornings usually start at 5:20, and I have alarms set until I leave the house at 7 a.m. As a practitioner of my preaching, I try my best not to go to bed too late either. So time was going to be my first obstacle to overcome. The way over that hurdle would be a realistic yet tight routine. Although, some in the productivity world separate routine from schedule, I needed to define and alter both. My morning routine would now include writing for an hour. I had to schedule it with my current morning routine of devotion and meditation, exercise, preparing my lunch, getting ready, and leaving on time. So I reworked my schedule, packed my lunch at night, put my clothes out at night, set a timer for the shower, eliminated the snooze button, and got up thirty minutes earlier but also went to bed an hour earlier each night.

The next obstacle would be getting everything done that I needed to accomplish each day. I had to examine the most important items on my plate over the upcoming weeks, so I had to take inventory and create new priorities that were in alignment with my new plan. Have you ever had so much going on, it seemed like one big hodgepodge of tasks and responsibilities? At times, that was me, and those were the times I felt drained and overwhelmed.

With so much to do, there's no realistic way to be wildly productive. The brain knows that. Remember, the brain really can only focus on one or two things at a time. The rest is flying around in your head like a tornado. In this flurry of thoughts, it's easy to let things fall through the cracks or lose sight of the goals ahead. This is a slippery slope because soon we can become even more slack rather than getting more done. The brain can't decide; it wants you to decide and stick to it. Rationalizations kick in: well I don't have what I need, I need more time, I need more money, I need more sleep, and I don't have a babysitter. All kinds of things get in the way, ready to rationalize your overwhelm and bail you out of this trap.

I had to determine the urgency from the important to the good ideas to the not-right-now by picking one or two goals for the week. I could take any tasks that related to that goal and sort through them to pick those with the least number of steps but the biggest results. The definite goal each week was to write 3,500 to 5,250 words in my book, no matter what.

I did just that and believe you me, it was tough at first. I chuckle now at the way my brain would automatically sort through its own database of excuses in the beginning. It was like someone speaking for me. "She's too tired, she needs more sleep, she's going to do it later, and so on." Day by day, it got easier. You know why? Because I was getting results. The brain likes results, or in other words, rewards. The brain is structured with a very simple concept yet complex neurohormonal system driven largely by the neurochemical dopamine, called the Brain Reward System or BRS, which connects and activates multiple areas of the brain including the pre-cortex, amygdala, hippocampus, and nucleus accumbens. If this all sounds like an intense episode of *Grey's Anatomy*, just remember, the brain has a lot to do with how consistent we are with anything, whether it's writing a book, making good food choices, losing weight, or studying. You name it. Results, winning, success, and accomplishments breed more of the same. Each day I reached the goal of 500 or more words for the allotted hour, the more motivated I was to tune out the distractions and do it over and over again.

Here's what I have used to train my personal success coaching clients. These are five strategies to gain more consistency in your life:

1. Have a new plan.

2. Push past the resistance to change.

3. Create and follow a new routine.

4. Adapt a "no excuses" policy.

5. Celebrate the small wins daily.

This is how I teach this concept. Go through the five-step strategy using sticky notes. Pick one priority or goal you have for the upcoming week. If your goal is to lose thirty pounds, let's look at what your goal is for just one week. Let's say you commit to lose two pounds in the upcoming week. What would you need to do consistently over the next seven days to make good on that commitment? Get very detailed in your description. Apply the questions: What? When? Where? Who? Which? How? Put each answer on a sticky note and place it beside the header sticky note with the primary goal. These surrounding detailed sticky notes will become the secondary goals; these will become your clear action steps. Follow them as if there is no other option. Really push beyond any excuse, obstacle, or barrier. In the pursuit of success of any type especially in weight loss, it's extremely important, in fact necessary, to master the principle of consistency. This life principle is not a sprint; this is a marathon. If you fall off track, don't go into a guilt trap. Get back on it, so you are more productive with your next set of goals.

We are what we repeatedly do. Excellence, then, is not an act, but a habit.

—Aristotle

Girl, Get Ready! Lesson #9:

The pace of your success depends on your consistency.

Action Step #9:

Applying this simple five-step strategy will help you pull the priorities out of the tornado and create an action plan that delivers results in a consistent and reliable way. Using this method across multiple areas will help you feel less overwhelmed and more successful, leading to strong, powerful emotions that serve you the most.

10

F the Ego

If you believe everything your ego tells you,
you're crazy.

Initially, I thought this would be the opening chapter of the book. After all, understanding the constructs of the ego would naturally give us invaluable insight into the remaining chapters of the book. However, I chose to put the ego here. Reflecting on the preceding chapters allows us to really see the ego in full swing in our everyday lives. This eventually makes sense in the end, much like the revealing, final moments of a mystery flick as the puzzle pieces begin to come together.

Ego is a word we hear pretty often, usually used to describe people who have negative or overbearing personalities. The word "ego" alone can be off-putting. If we go back into the early years of development of this ageless theory, Dr. Sigmund Freud, a brilliant, eccentric psychologist, posed the ideology of three distinctly interactive representatives that characterize Freud's model of the psyche. These are widely known as id, ego, and superego. The id is the primitive and instinctual part of the mind that contains sexual and aggressive drives and hidden memories, the superego operates as a moral conscience, and the ego is the realistic part that mediates between the desires of the id and the superego.

Without a full, advanced psychology lecture, let's skip right to why this ego thing matters in this conversation. See, ego is where the majority of us spend our waking hours in our headspace. Throughout the day, we are thinking, decision-making, choosing, and functioning inside of the reasoning of our reality as we see it. Based on what that part of the psyche does, being in ego most of the time is neither good nor bad. The main thing is to just know that being in a constant state of awareness is how we make good on what could otherwise seemingly be considered bad.

Now that I've gotten your attention, let's go to the science of it. Don't check out because you need to hear this. It's not a sermon; it's a lecture. Take the information, study it, and use it for the test. Your brain has a center called the amygdala. Let's just assign it as a "him." We'll call him Mr. Feel Good, and let's give him his props, Mr. Feel Great! The amygdala is critical for opioid-mediated binge eating of fat (Will, Matthew J.; Franzblau, Emily B.; Kelley, Ann E.; NeuroReport. 15(12):1857–1860, August 26, 2004).

Here's the CliffNotes version for the non-science enthusiasts: So, there's a place in the brain that longs to be satisfied. No matter what, it is always ready to go off the deep end and is often the cause for frantic, anxious behaviors, getting in your feelings, and losing control. This very same center lives in the neighborhood of the appetite control center and can easily influence the appetite to be increased or in some cases decreased. If and when this happens, typically, the emotions win first, then the makeup session follows. This can be an ongoing cycle until something interrupts this.

One of the most difficult parts about the ego, the amygdala, and the emotional rants is that it all seems so real. So, it's important to recognize that the brain holds the physiologic ability to govern memory, planning, calculating, concentrating, analyzing, and comprehension. The mind, as a function of the brain's performance capacity, takes over with thinking, habits, behaviors, and conjuring up scenarios, reactions, and other expressions. The ego fits right in here, with feeding emotions from a position of judgment and self-orientation. When the ego is involved, it's the "all about me," self-centered likes, wants, desires, and more. This will create a problem-focused, fear-based, irrational, close-minded way of functioning, which is a setup for poor decision-making.

Biologically speaking, there are two categories where the ego can be like gasoline to a flame: eating and sex. It is incredibly important to know this and to learn how to take clear actions that promote more critical thinking and less emotional decision-making. This approach is mission driven, empathic, logical, rational, objective, and data-oriented, open-minded, and solution-focused.

<u>Girl, Get Ready! Lesson #10:</u>

We can't afford to operate and run off fleeting emotions. It's essential to F the ego in order to power ahead in the transformation journey.

<u>Action Step #10:</u>

Look back at the last five decisions you made about eating (or anything for that matter). Compare and contrast how you make decisions.

Body

11

Metabolism: This Is Amazing

*A healthy metabolism is like a well-oiled machine;
it requires regular maintenance.*

Metabolism is everything. This is the lynchpin of the whole weight thing. Consider this process the control center of anything you consume. When you take in energy—which is in plain terms, food—your system has to process it and decide what to do with the byproducts once it enters the body. The whole cascade begins before you actually put a morsel into your mouth. However, we'll cover that a little later in this section.

To begin, let's take a trip down Bodyworks Lane to help make sense of this word you probably see and hear all the time. From infomercials to drugstore shelves, metabolism is usually a wastebasket term that few people really understand. Without bringing back dreaded memories of biochemistry, let me simplify this for you. No, you won't need a pen and paper, just read carefully and use your imagination. Think for a moment of what is going on internally in your body. Your initial thought might be that you're sleepy, hungry, or achy from an intense workout. But let's think a little deeper, getting beyond the surface level of your conscious thoughts or feelings. We'll take a closer look at what's going on in the trillions of cells that make up the human body.

If you could examine the inside of any of these tiny cells, you'll discover a busy hub of hundreds of workstations similar to a manufacturing facility with thousands of assembly workers, conveyor belts, production lines, and supply transporters, buzzing and moving about twenty-four hours a day. Think of the energy that is required to simply keep the lights on, let alone what it takes to keep every single element functioning like a well-oiled machine. To drive home the point, think of it like this; you could be fast asleep or working in the middle of the day, kickboxing in a gym, or vegging out watching Netflix, but at any given time, energy is being used, converted, transferred, or stored inside your cells with a flurry of ongoing chemical reactions, taking place to keep you viable and functional.

This collection of reactions that manage energy (think food) follow one of two pathways: breaking down (catabolic) or building up (anabolic) functions. There are two very critical processes that are essential to life on Earth. These are the steps that lead to the breakdown and the buildup of sugars (glucose). We'll explore this concept further in the chapter. For now, just know that what happens at the cellular level generates the overall metabolic ability at the organ level, and of course, you recall that organs make up systems, which depend on a robust, healthy, and high-performing metabolism to carry out daily functions, process food intake, and balance energy, ultimately determining if you lose, gain, or maintain weight at any given time.

But before we move on, you may have a few questions in mind. For example, does the metabolism vary from person to person? The answer is of course, it definitely varies between people. Since metabolism shifts and changes depending on the conditions of the organism, the human body can speed up and slow down the rates of different chemical processes and reactions at any given time. When that happens, the inherent regulations within those two pathways mentioned earlier are for the sole purpose of maintaining homeostasis. In short, this happens to keep the body from making wide swings from one state to another.

Your next question is probably something like, "Does weight have an impact on metabolism?" You're getting good at this! That biology is coming right back to you. Yes, weight can affect metabolism, and metabolism can affect weight. It's one of those age-old questions like which comes first, the chicken or the egg? We won't deliberate that argument. It really doesn't matter so much as knowing that the two are closely interdependent.

While weight is influenced by metabolism and vice versa, it certainly isn't the only factor that does so. A person's activity levels, hormone levels, age, energy intake, and overall health can also impact metabolism. For example, you could have an illness and whether you're sick with the flu for a week or have been diagnosed with a chronic condition such as polycystic ovarian syndrome, several things can occur in the body to throw off your usual or native body functions. In the case of the flu, your energy utilization may be higher due to the effects of a fever. In the latter case, one or more of your hormones is producing more or less than normal, causing a hormone imbalance. In either case, your cellular and eventually overall metabolism would either downregulate or upregulate as needed. Now that you have a general understanding of the ins and outs of metabolism, let's move on to the next "M" of weight loss.

Girl, Get Ready! Lesson #11:

Healthy metabolism is dynamic; it is not fixed; it regulates changes based on the body's demand.

Action Step #11:

1. Get on the scale and record your weight EVERY SINGLE DAY for ten days in a row.

2. Journal what you consume (meaning anything you eat or drink) for each of these ten days.

3. Compare each day to see what changes you notice in your weight.

12

Macronutrients: Mistakes I've Seen Made Over and Over Again

If muscle weighs more than fat,
why do you see more fat than muscle?

Now that you understand some basics about the inner workings of the metabolic system, let's add some meat to the bones. (Yes, pun intended!) By now, you've probably become broadly familiar with the terms macronutrients, or "macros" for the well-versed or in many cases the not so well-versed groupies who have jumped on the next bandwagon smokin' in search of a thin, lean oasis. Here, we'll go somewhere in between. You don't need to have a PhD in nutrition to effectively develop winning meal plans and navigate grocery store aisles. Likewise, you don't want to go about it like a newbie who's following a plan found in a magazine in the checkout lane but don't really have a clue as to why you're actually eating that way and what results you can expect.

Macronutrients refer to a class of foods that are required in relatively large quantities in order to provide calories and therefore energy to the body to carry out daily functions. There are three main foods that fall into that category: proteins, carbohydrates, and fats. I also like to include two other categories, fiber and water. These two are essential macronutrients that are not manufactured must be consumed and are critical for survival.

First, we should clarify what large quantities mean. In short, large is in regard to the sizable amount of the nutrients available in the amounts needed to do a specific job. In this case, large amounts (on the order of hundreds and thousands) are required to provide the calories or energy for the human body to function in its usual capacity. It is key to remember these six characteristics of macronutrients:

1. Essential in large amounts

2. Should be eaten in proper proportions

3. Excessive intake can lead to diseases, worsen health conditions, or make one more prone to illness

4. Makes up the bulk of the foods we eat

5. Determines the calories we consume

6. Provides the nutrient substances needed for growth, metabolism, and body functions

On the flip side of that, micronutrients are required in smaller amounts (micro and milligrams) to carry out their primary job, which is to support enzyme production and cellular functions. Think of it like this: enzymes are like little enhancers that help things to break down and become smaller, more user friendly, and digestible versions of the original particle. So, there are nutrients needed to help those enzymes do their job. These are called micronutrients. We'll talk more about those in the next chapter. Let's talk about macronutrients.

PROTEINS

Proteins are made up of multiple combinations of smaller functional nutrients called amino acids. The most important roles of proteins are to

- Build muscle
- Repair damaged tissue and cells
- Maintain a healthy robust immune system
- Produce hormones

When you consume food, you should be thinking about what results this food will produce in your body. This is a more valuable reasoning tool than making food choices based on moods, feelings, tastes, and other fleeting thoughts. When thinking of protein intake, think about what exactly this food will cause to happen in your body. Below are the key functions of proteins expected once you take a bite of that juicy steak or bowl of tofu.

Protein functions:

- Makes up four calories per gram of protein (believe it or not, at the same rate as carbohydrates)
- Satisfies hunger because it is the most filling macronutrient
- Reduces cravings
- Increases metabolism
- Keeps blood sugar (glucose) balanced

CARBOHYDRATES

Carbohydrates, semi-affectionately referred to as "carbs," get a bad rap in the diet world. Before we go by hearsay and join the camp, let's visit a few of the key roles of carbohydrates. I think you'll understand why we shouldn't be so hard on this high-energy nutrient and also why it's important to know your stuff when it comes to carbohydrates, so you avoid the common pitfalls of carbohydrate metabolism. The most important roles of carbohydrates are to

- Provide immediate calories as fuel for activity
- Store energy for later
- Help preserve muscle composition
- Fuel exercise performance

Now, are you starting to see why carbs aren't so bad after all? Carbohydrates are critically necessary for every cell in our bodies, especially brain cells. Similar to proteins, carbohydrates come in different shapes and sizes to best accommodate the many jobs that they must perform. That's why there are so many differences between the carbs we eat.

One main difference is simple versus complex. A basic explanation is that complex carbs are bigger and take longer to break down, so they hang around in our systems, keeping us with a steady supply of energy for a prolonged period of time. Simple carbohydrates stop by for the party, make a big splash, get your body all hyped up, and then bail out, leaving you feeling drained and washed out once they're gone. Go to www.girlgetreadybook.com to see a sample chart of how we source our energy throughout the day.

The other way to look at this is based on a concept called glycemic index. All that means is that we can look at carbohydrates in categories based on how fast and how high they cause our blood sugars to spike once we've eaten them. Low glycemic foods gradually increase sugars to a reasonable level for sustained use, high glycemic foods increase our blood sugar rapidly, and any unused sugar gets stored as fat after about an hour or so. So, it becomes obvious what the better choice is. Remember, we are starting to look at food choices based on their function, not our feelings. The Harvard Medical School publication has a great article and table that describe this concept in great detail and can be found by going to the resource document at www.girlgetreadybook.com.

Carbohydrate functions:

- Provide energy for muscles for activity
- Regulates blood sugar
- Preserves protein use
- Aids in digestion

Needless to say, carbohydrates need not stand out as the black sheep of the macronutrient family; however, we do have to understand how to make these nutrients work to our advantage and not to our disadvantage.

FATS

Until recently, fats have also been deemed the nutritional stepchild in the dietary world. In the past, fats have been associated with heart disease, kidney problems, and high cholesterol. In some ways, that distinction still holds true; however, we have learned, and in my experience, the right fats in the diet can work wonders for the metabolism, weight loss, and essential body functions. The most important roles of fats are to

- Provide essential fatty acids, which the body cannot do by itself
- Store energy for use when protein and carbohydrate sources are unavailable in the needed supply
- Regulate body temperature
- Provide structure to cells, especially in the nerves and brain

Wouldn't you say that was pretty important stuff? We need fats to thrive. However, it's the right amounts and the right type of fats that make the difference between using their fat superpowers for good versus evil. To make this plain and clear, look below for the key functions of fats.

Fat functions:

- Helps the body absorb essential vitamins like A, D, E, and K
- Suppresses hunger between meals
- Assists with hormone balance
- Enhances elasticity and functioning of artery walls

Fats come to the rescue in many ways, and they can do so in double the capacity as carbohydrates or proteins with nine calories per gram compared to four. For more examples of best animal and plant protein sources, simple versus complex, low glycemic versus high glycemic carbohydrates, and top choice fats, check out www.girlgetreadybook.com.

That was a long chapter I know, but we had to get some key points established. Now, we can move on.

Girl, Get Ready! Lesson #12:

Macronutrients need to shift based on what's required. Don't get stuck on a formula to determine what you need. Sometimes it's best to learn to listen to your body.

Action Step #12:

Complete a 24-hour "Food Recall." Track every bite or sip you have consumed in the past 24-hour period. Note which foods made you function the best.

13

Micronutrients: Okay, I've Got to Get This Right

Big things come in small packages.

Micronutrients are just as they sound: nutrients that are required in much smaller quantities to keep our bodies in serious motion with optimal vitality. In short, micronutrients are another name for vitamins and minerals. These are often significantly overlooked in the popular diet and the weight loss theories that we see come and go. We'll break down just a few important points. If you understand and execute these SIX simple principles, you're well on your way.

1. **Supply and Demand:** Micronutrients enable the body to produce enzymes, hormones, and other substances essential for nearly every function of the body. When these are in abundant supply, you can do all of those things efficiently, effectively, and consistently. When vitamins and minerals are in limited or short supply, those functions suffer greatly and result in a system that's working harder and is not as productive, which can eventually lead to burnout or dysfunction.

2. **Hide and Go Seek:** Vitamins and minerals are best sourced from food, so we're told. Yet, some foods

don't have the nutrients we think they do because of how food in the world is produced, transported, and stored these days. The other issue is that some foods require us to eat so much of it to get those tiny amounts of nutrients that it's either unrealistic, unlikely, undesirable, or unhelpful to consume so many extra calories in the exchange. For example, be careful eating bananas for the potassium! The average adult should consume 3,500 to 4,000 mg of potassium each day. The average banana has about 420 mg of potassium and 105 calories each. That means if you were using bananas as a go-to to tank up on this important nutrient, you would need to eat about nine bananas. This is roughly 950 calories, of which 98 percent is made up of carbohydrates. I know the math can be confusing. Don't worry, we'll cover more about this in later sections. You can get more information on the website, www.girlgetreadybook.com.

3. **Consumption versus Absorption:** Just because you take in vitamins and minerals doesn't mean they're doing the job they should be doing. Vitamins and minerals can easily be a part of your intake but miss prime opportunities for absorption if digestive tract conditions aren't just right. Generally speaking, vitamins and minerals will begin maximum absorption in the small intestine. If you miss this small window of opportunity, you may be getting only a fraction of what you think you are despite regular use. This is

usually because of one of three things: health of the gut, competition with other things, or quality of the supplement.

4. **Health of the Gut:** The gut, i.e., the digestive tract, starts with the mouth and goes for miles to the very bottom of your large intestines called the anus, which leads back to the outward world. When the gut is healthy and at its best, there's a strong, tight barrier in the intestinal lining supported by a symbiotic, balanced environment of beneficial bacteria that aid in digestion and allow no interference of other stuff that takes away from the system. Sometimes, processed ingredients, environmental byproducts, medications, illness, intolerances, genetics, and stress can be very disruptive to the digestive organs leading to a sick, poorly functioning, low-absorbing system. At that point, vitamins and minerals are lost and deficiencies begin to show up in subtle ways and often go undiagnosed for years.

5. **Us versus Them:** As mentioned, food allergies, sensitivities, and intolerances can occur for many reasons. Some of it is genetic predisposition, but a lot of it is because of the immune system, which by the way is in large part influenced by the gut. Many different preservatives and chemicals used to grow food can be the very things that jeopardize vitamin, mineral, and nutrient absorption. Plus, beware of what I call "big box" vitamins; you know the ones on the shelves

in major large chain stores where popular marketing has earned them a place in the spotlight. Yet the mass production of low quality supplements full of preservatives, fillers, and dyes can leave you worse off than you started.

6. **Natural versus Synthetic:** The question is often asked about the best way to get vitamins, minerals, and nutrients to benefit the body. At some point, the issue of whether supplements really work, and then the question of natural versus synthetic, will arise. What's the difference, and does it really matter? In my experience and philosophy, natural and synthetic are sometimes more useful as marketing buzzwords. Natural is a matter of interpretation, and synthetic isn't always so bad.

Of course, I recommend as a rule of thumb, the closer a food is to its natural state of evolution, the better it is for you. I also realize we live in an industrialized world and that changes a lot of what we experience when it comes to purity and integrity of foods. I don't like it, but that's the way it is.

In summary, micronutrients are small yet complex to some extent. When it comes to food, the cleanest food with the least chemical exposure eaten sooner rather than later once it leaves the earth supplies the most micronutrients. The key to supplements is to get the purest products, the best routes of absorption, and the most functional versions.

Go to www.girlgetreadybook.com for some of my favorite healthy food sources and my preferred brands of supplements.

Girl, Get Ready! Lesson #13:

Carrying excess weight robs the body of important vitamins, minerals, and nutrients that are needed for a healthy metabolism.

Action Step #13:

Using the food recall list, research to see what and how many nutrients are in those foods. Find out which nutrients can be found in some of your favorite foods at girlgetreadybook.com

---

14

Muscle: There's More to This Than I Thought

Don't overcomplicate it.

After a hefty talk about macros and micros, you're sufficiently prepared to be briefed on one of the MVP's of metabolism: muscle. Muscle, a complex network of dense fibrous tissue, has three different types and three distinct functions. I'll give you a super-condensed version of this concept straight out of Anatomy and Physiology 101.

Muscles are categorized as either cardiac, smooth, or skeletal. Cardiac muscle is self-explanatory; it's the primary tissue type of the heart. It serves as a conduit of electrical impulses to keep the heart beating in synchrony and pumping with finesse. Cardiac muscle, though involuntary and operating outside of our control, is very sensitive to stress, neurotransmitters, hormones, and micronutrients.

Smooth muscle is also considered involuntary muscle that generally serves as a lining of blood vessels, organs, and major passageways. This muscle type ensures that our lungs breathe, bowels move, kidneys filter, and the reproductive system reproduces.

Skeletal muscle is voluntary in action. Attached to bones, ligaments, tendons, and other connective tissue, skeletal muscle results in the movement of our bodies, protects organs, and produces heat. Skeletal muscle carries out very important work when it comes to motion, but more importantly for weight loss, its potential for energy exchange is major.

This is where we tie in macronutrients, micronutrients, and metabolism. You've heard it said that muscle burns more than fat. There's some truth to that on the order of about three times more calories are used by muscle compared to fat. This is especially relevant to at-rest energy use. But, for the sake of this discussion, let's focus on the burn, not the comparison.

Five key points to remember about muscle and weight loss:

1. Muscle is made up mainly of various complex proteins.

2. Muscle uses all three macronutrients for fuel: proteins, carbohydrates, and fats.

3. Muscle burns or utilizes three times the calories that fat does, especially at rest.

4. Muscle increases strength and agility.

5. Good muscle tone prevents injury and promotes flexibility.

Building and maintaining good muscle structure is an important goal in weight loss and long-term weight control. Scientifically, there's no one-size-fits-all to muscle mass goals, testing, or percentages. Women will average about 26 to 31 percent depending on age, height, ethnicity, and more. Men will average about 31 to 44 percent with similar variations. The overall goal is to continue to build and maintain lean muscle and reduce body fat, which tends to be a more accurate marker to follow.

Girl, Get Ready! Lesson #14:

Decreasing body fat is the key priority followed by increasing muscle structure for successful weight loss. Everybody has a "six pack." You just have to eliminate the fat that's covering it up to see it.

Action Step #14:

Determine what your fat and muscle percentages are by consulting with your doctor or weight loss professional if needed.

15

Movement: Oh, So That's Why

Show me your moves.

Now, you're starting to see the pieces of the weight loss puzzle coming together. Movement is the next step in the natural progression of things. I like to use the term "movement" as a catchall word to include any type of physical activity, exercise, workouts, conditioning, or other forms of exertion that result in the expenditure of energy. Whether working in your yard or working out at the gym, it all adds up, and the more of it you do, the better off you are with controlling your weight. Did you notice I said controlling your weight? Yes, that was intentional. I find in my practice and in my experience, well-meaning people tend to have very lofty expectations of a 30-minute exercise routine. I usually hear people lament that they have been working out for months and haven't lost a single pound. In fact, in many cases, they may have even gained pounds. Whether working out solo or paying big bucks for a personal trainer, the results tend to be very similar. I can tell you time and time again, I have clients who are at their wits' end because they have worked their knees into a state of shock, run enough miles to travel two states over, and still can't get their scales to show even the slightest glimpse of a reward.

I have to convince them that I can help them get the weight off with a fraction of the exhaustion and stress if they will only yield to the process. Through years of doing this work and thousands of patients I've assisted on the path to successful and lasting weight loss, there are four crucial things to understand:

1. Exercise alone will not result in significant weight loss.

2. The right exercise for the right outcome at the right phase of weight loss is imperative.

3. There is such a thing as too much exercise.

4. The best forms of movement happen continuously, consistently, and correctly.

Let's sort through those.

Exercise alone will not result in lasting weight loss. I have a saying, and you've likely heard it before. You can't outrun your fork. In our society, there's a tendency to eat whatever we want and add a 30-minute workout three times a week to our calendar and sit back to watch the magic happen. That fallacy has resulted in overcrowded gyms full of people who are still struggling to lose weight. Just a few doors down and a parking lot over, there are jam-packed restaurants filled with people enjoying meals they didn't prepare, with ingredients they can hardly pronounce, and of course, the tasty beverages they order by the refills to wash down their calorie-dense, nutrient-poor meals, in some cases multiple times a day.

Exercise becomes the Hail Mary fourth quarter long shot that many hope will erase the detriments of "good to you food" in large quantities and in any combination. My friends, exercise will not save you. We've got to have a more solid plan A or C because plan B is played out.

Next, doing random exercises and workouts for the sake of checking a box, hanging out at the gym, or to lose excess weight will seldom work in your favor. No, I'm not trying to talk you out of working out. I am trying to talk you into working out with purpose and with strategy. You see, there are a variety of activities that, when done properly and for an adequate period of time and in a well-constructed pattern, can be your best defense to compliment a good offense (eating to lose).

I require all of my patients to undergo a professional fitness assessment, so we can get a sense of their goals, strengths, weak spots, any injury prone areas or previous injuries, previous surgeries, or anatomical defects from birth. For long-range success, a well-devised strategic fitness plan is just what this doctor orders.

There is such a thing as too much exercise, to the extent that it stresses the body rather than helps it. This causes inflammation and sends out stress signals that will alert the body to hold on to fat, release toxins, and short-circuit valuable hormone production. There's nothing more disheartening for me than to hear the horror stories of obese and morbidly obese patients who have literally been dragged through the mud, yelled at, criticized, scoffed at, injured, and left disappointed and distraught as a result of workout routines that frankly weren't right for them in the first place. You have probably been one of them at some point on your wellness journey.

When it comes to exercise for weight loss, I don't suggest you go with conventional wisdom or pop-up "get fit quick" schemes. There is no reason to rush the process and risk a setback. This is one of those times less can be more. Resist the urge to overdo it. I know you may be tempted by others around you or determined to work off that bowl of ice cream and cookies, but abruptly pushing yourself beyond reasonable limits can backfire, leaving you worse off than when you started.

The most profitable approach to exercise for my clients is to work on getting the weight down 10 to 15 percent first, then complete a professional fitness assessment, and then begin a stepwise fitness regimen that builds up over time and is in concert with the intended goals of each phase of active weight loss and then compatible with maintenance. The pillars we teach for a high-performing fitness regimen are:

- Continuously – Using physical activity and movement each day is not solely to lose weight. It is to train the metabolism and the body to create a certain yield of calorie use all day long. In this case, I emphasize doing things you enjoy, so you are drawn to it instead of dreading it. In my case, I love walking. I believe if time allowed and weather permitted, I could walk eight hours a day. Now, finding an activity you enjoy that much may be a stretch but find a few things that you look forward to doing each day. At least a couple should be home friendly, so you have ready-to-go default options in the event you can't get to a gym or the weather doesn't work with your original plans.

- Correctly – Get help with new routines and activities, especially weight training and running. Some things may seem like a no-brainer, but as products and equipment have been improved through advanced engineering, they may not be as intuitive as they once were or the last time you used them. Similarly, as we get older, there are differences in our body mechanics that can heavily influence our abilities to exercise or engage in physical movement safely. I recommend the fitness assessment and a graduated program for those over forty who are resuming or starting a new plan. Even if you were a former athlete, runner, swimmer, boxer, tennis player, or golfer, there are things to consider when you have been out of the swing of things (pun intended). One of the biggest mistakes I see is that we're so eager to engage in the activity we don't give proper time and attention to the practice of stretching the body before and after the activity. Stretching should occur every single time you get up and move about. In our age of sitting more than ever, muscles, tendons, and ligaments get contracted, tight, and resistant. Stretching helps to reduce injury, improve flexibility, and avoid excessive soreness.

- Consistency – That which you do often, you do better. That's one of my favorite mantras. In this case, making exercise, daily movement, and physical activity a part of your daily life is better for your heart, lungs, brain, joints, and overall health. This helps keep your baseline metabolism active, engaged, and nimble. I instruct all of my clients to look at their calendars and place standing appointments every day for their activity, and then set reminders and alerts for those appointments and let nothing get in the way of that plan. Set up your life to honor yourself and your commitment to yourself. Not only do I recommend daily exercise (yes, seven days a week), but I also recommend spurts of movement incorporated into your day, especially for those who work from home or have desk jobs with very limited movement. Then there are my clients who have jobs that require lots of physical labor, yet they still struggle with their weight. There has to be a new activity incorporated to balance that work activity. Usually, I find it to be the exact opposite of what they do every day.

In summary, movement is the cornerstone of optimal health and well-being. The benefits of movement are undeniable. Having a solid plan and sufficient preparation is a setup for success.

Girl, Get Ready! Lesson #15:

Movement is the cornerstone of optimum health and well-being.

Action Step #15:

Make an activity calendar that incorporates some of your favorite things to do. Some examples could be swimming, rollerblading, or yoga.

16

Meals: Where Do I Start?

Home-cooked meals matter.

We started the last chapter with the clear declaration that exercise matters, but food matters more. There are so many details when it comes to food, meals, snacks, menus, meal prep, the drive-thru, grocery store runs, food delivery services—I get it. There's so much to take into consideration when it comes to developing eating habits that work for us and not against us. When it comes to weight loss, there's no doubt that eating is the part the majority of people struggle with the most. And when I say struggle, that can mean a number of things; however, in this context, it means in my experience, people find the most challenges with mastering eating in these three areas: nutritionally, logistically, and behaviorally (which we will cover in the next chapter).

Nutritionally speaking, when it comes to eating and particularly eating meals, there are a few common mistakes I see all the time. Well, actually there are a lot of them, but if you master these three strategies, you're ready to turn things around for the good.

1. Make your meals at home.

   a. Don't leave your health up to strangers.

b. Learn how to cook foods that are easy, appealing, and tasty.

c. Don't overthink or "overfeel" when it comes to meals; use an eating guide.

2. Maximize your results by eating foods and meals that align with your goals.

a. If your goal is more energy, eat foods that are light and high in antioxidants like colorful vegetables and fruits. Steer clear of foods high in carbohydrates; those will zap your energy fast.

b. If your goal is to sleep well, eat small evening meals and cut off eating at least three hours before bedtime, and avoid heavy sauces, spicy foods, and red meat in the evenings.

c. If your goal is to lose weight, follow your meal plan, eat with your health in mind, lean toward protein and fresh foods, and avoid large portions of food. Don't eat until you're stuffed; instead, eat the portion allotted for that meal.

3. Use the following data to guide how you will eat each week.

a. Measure your blood pressure.

b. Weigh yourself.

c. Check your blood sugar.

Logistically, in other words, what does it take for you to control what you eat, when you eat, and how much you eat? The details of logistics are the stuff that can make or break the best of intentions. I work with busy professionals, entrepreneurs, corporate leaders, and public and political figures, and this one is always a big challenge to overcome for weight loss success.

Mastering logistics requires creativity, innovation, risk, and discipline. I always marvel at the fact that most of my clients are accustomed to years of accomplishments using those very same qualities, except when it comes to eating for success. Acknowledging this can be very disheartening for someone who is often in the winning seat. This often poses itself as a threat and can become a rigid barrier to overcome.

This 3-step process can help set up a game plan to apply those same winning principles to this new game of controlling eating patterns, no matter what the circumstances.

1. Control what you eat by having your food plan tight. I usually recommend taking your food with you every day. That means you have to master the meals part we spoke of earlier, which requires a strategy for shopping, cooking, and prepping.

   Some creative ways to do that are to:

   - Schedule a shop day, cook day, and prep day. By breaking the steps down, you may find it much easier to take on each task separately.

- Set up a virtual play date with friends or family to cook or prep together. You will look forward to spending time with people you enjoy while you both invest in your health.

- Join a recipe group. You rotate who picks recipes for the week and also create a grocery list at the same time. All you have to do is grab the items, so half the work is done.

- Use online grocery shopping, pickup, and delivery options to save time and keep you from buying stuff that's not on your list. The software is so good these days that it remembers previous shopping items and makes it super easy to fill your basket with good food, save time, and is something you can schedule regularly on your calendar instead of running out of food and rushing to the store or grabbing a quick bite out instead.

- Join a Community Supported Agriculture (CSA) program. This is a great way to provide you and your family with healthy, usually organic, and local produce. A CSA box may be available as a monthly subscription, which brings to your fingertips various locally grown, seasonal fruits and vegetables at an affordable price.

- Hire a private chef. This is a great alternative to eating out and allows you to better manage your food selections, quality, and nutritional value that supports your weight loss goals without compromising taste or time. Believe it or not, this can actually save you money in the long run.

- Use a meal delivery service. These services are becoming quite popular, and the prices are very competitive, allowing you to save money compared to eating out or picking up restaurant food. You know well in advance what you will have, and you can easily plan your healthy, fresh, ready-to-go meals in no time.

2. Control when you eat by scheduling your meals and snacks like you schedule your meetings with your boss, your team, or your highest-paying client. In other words, make it a priority and stick to it. Now, the art and science of when to eat and what to eat can be complicated, and that's where I recommend you get with a specialty-trained, weight loss physician or other credible health and wellness professional who has extensive experience to really begin to determine the best eating strategies to result in boosting your metabolism, losing weight, increasing energy, and maximizing the benefits of your physical activity. I spend a lot of time with my clients in this area. In fact, it's a very important part of the customized plans I develop for my clients. There's no doubt that eating the right foods at the right times is one of the key parts of a successful weight loss plan.

3. Control how much you eat by knowing how much you need to consume per day, per meal, and per serving. While these may vary some from day to day, it's generally not going to vary by much. Depending on your weight loss goals and your physiological needs, I usually have patients eat based on the data we use. That data comes from the scale, your blood sugar, your blood pressure, physical messages, and what activities you have to do each day (work out, yard work, labor intensive job, desk work, lazy day, etc.). This is a primary reason I insist my clients weigh themselves daily. We have to have the data for decision-making. Just like you check your bank account to determine how much you can spend each day or check your vehicle's gas gauge to see how many miles you can go before fueling up again, you should check the scale to confirm your eating plans for the day, the week, and the month. Some people rely on calories, some on macros, and some on a combination of both to actually determine how much food to consume. Either way, how much is an integral part of weight management. Again, I suggest getting with a professional to help figure that out. There's no one-size-fits-all here.

Girl, Get Ready! Lesson #16:

You have to know and control what goes in your body in order to establish a healthy and robust metabolism.

Action Step #16

Create a seven-day meal plan using the information from the chapters. Click on www.girlgetreadybook.com for a sample meal plan.

Mindless Eating: Where Does That Come From?

I'm always amazed at women who carry expensive handbags, yet feed themselves cheap food.

We covered two key areas of mastering meals, or eating in general for that matter, in the last chapter: nutritional and logistical. Now, let's cover the final area, behavioral mastery. Behavior is a huge contributor to our eating habits. Just like anything else, we generally describe behavior as good or bad, acceptable or unacceptable, or some similar dichotomous assignment. In a simple fashion, human behavior can best be described as the full range of physical and emotional ways of functioning that humans engage in and how they conduct themselves in their lives biologically, socially, and intellectually. Behaviors can be shaped and influenced by rapport, culture, attitudes, emotions, ethics, values, authority, persuasion, coercion, and genetics. With that being established, the behavioral side of eating is a complex collection of experiences that we draw on to make decisions and choices about our whole approach to eating and to food in general. We covered a good bit of this in the first section of this book, but now, we can add another layer to connect the dots even further.

Many food behaviors begin in childhood, and some may argue in utero or prior to even being born. If we take that into consideration along with all of the food experiences that occur over the span of childhood to adulthood, it's clear that we carry a lot of those influences into the habits we create around food. For the sake of this chapter, let's focus on those habits, particularly the habit of mindless eating. Mindless eating is described as the practice of consuming foods or beverages without giving consideration or regard to the circumstance related to or leading up to the consumption. In plain terms, you may have heard this described as "eating with your eyes and not your stomach" or "head hunger versus true hunger." These are discoveries I have often with my clients. In many cases, people have become conditioned to eat, drink, and be merry without thinking before choosing or going along with the flow of their environment. There are three habits that I have seen in combination over the years in my profession.

1. Adults' eating patterns are largely driven by their childhood upbringing around eating. Now, interestingly enough, people outgrow a lot of things related to childhood like bedwetting, the desire to become a mermaid when they grow up, or the belief in Santa, the Easter Bunny, and the Tooth Fairy. Yet, when it comes to food beliefs, they persist, often in a pervasive and subconscious manner. Our palates are older, but our brains are stuck in a time warp. That is one area we really have to go back to dissect, understand,

and reckon with. I often spend a sizable part of coaching going back in time in order to make strides in the present.

2. Eating to the point of no return. Over the years, most of my clients have quite likely spent their entire lives overriding the physiological cues of hunger and satiety. In other words, eating food when not hungry or continuing to eat more food when the early signs of fullness have kicked in, yet these signs are ignored. This is one that I often hear from adults about how these practices were started as infants when being fed infant formula from a baby bottle. Every wince or whimper was met with a bottle being shoved into their mouths. Whether true in childhood or self-indulged in adolescence as a coping mechanism, eating or resorting to comfort eating during stressful times in adulthood, consumption of food without regard to its impact on the body, and the inability to control it is a destructive habit that undermines the most sophisticated plans for weight control. The bigger problem is that once this happens, it generates a vicious cycle of reinforcing actions both physical and psychological that are seldom resolved without legitimate support and ongoing professional input.

3. Environmental cues influence eating choices. And according to Brian Wansink, Professor and Director of the famed Cornell University Food and Brand Lab, where he is a leading expert in changing eating

behavior, "We are discovering that there are a lot of mindless habits that go into eating. But, we're also finding that these mindless eating habits can easily be changed, not by education, but by essentially changing the environment." Likewise, in my work with clients, I firmly assert that when there are poor options, people will make poor choices, and when there are excellent options, people are more likely to make excellent choices. But, this is true only in the absence of poor choices. See when they both coexist, the likelihood of poor selections is far greater than when there are only healthy, high-quality selections available. In my work with clients, I urge them to control their narrative by setting themselves up for success and eliminating all sabotaging options from the equation. Now, if only it were that simple, you probably wouldn't be reading this book. The moral of this story is that the more structures you put in place to be successful, the more likely you are to become successful. So, every little bit counts. Never underestimate the power of baby steps because enough of them put together can lead to the giant leap we often only dream of.

4. The opposite of mindless eating is mindful eating. All that means is that you put structures, strategies, and tools in place to carefully contemplate everything you eat and choose from an informed, intentional, and goals-oriented position. As simple as that may sound,

that is something that must be taught and reinforced repeatedly.

Over the years, I have used similar theory to help clients through rough behavioral and psychological patches when it comes to weight loss, healthy living, and wellness-based practices. In my practice, I have developed my own terminology for teaching people how to lose weight and keep it off by teaching people how to eat. Using a host of data collected from personal history, psychosocial evaluations, and medical assessments of clients I've worked with over the years, I have used my proven methodology to introduce the concept of Strategic Eating. This can be taught at any age to anyone ready to take more personalized yet guided strategies through individual and group coaching.

Using the information presented up until this point gives you a lot of tools in your toolbox to help you devise simple yet solid steps toward getting the weight down with sound, consistent lifestyle changes that you can follow and build upon for the long haul.

Girl, Get Ready! Lesson #17:

Mindful eating requires you to be present in your goal and your "why."

Action Step #17:

For the next seven days, eat your meals without any distractions, meaning no TV, no computer, and no cellphone, etc. Observe your thoughts while you enjoy your meal.

18

Medications: Problem or Solution?

Medicine should be a bridge, not a crutch.

I tucked this chapter in here because I get a lot of questions from doctors, students I mentor, and clients about medications and weight loss. In some cases, the question is, do some medications cause weight gain or difficulty with weight loss? In other cases, I'm asked if medications help with weight loss and whether they are safe. The next most common question is, how long should one take medications for weight loss, and do they create a dependency? So, here are the answers I usually give to my clients:

1. There are a number of medications that I look for when seeing new clients for weight loss. To simplify things, I'll put them here by class and most commonly prescribed in the class.

   - Beta blockers – usually for blood pressure and heart conditions, migraines and anxiety; some examples are Metoprolol, Atenolol, and Propranolol.
   - Psychotropics/antidepressants – usually used for psychiatric conditions like schizophrenia and similar conditions such as bipolar disorder, depression, and anxiety.

- Steroids – used for a variety of conditions like rheumatoid arthritis, lupus, sarcoidosis, connective tissue disorders, and lung disorders to name a few; usually Prednisone, Prednisolone, and Methylprednisolone are prescribed.

- Hormone therapy – In the case of birth control and hormone imbalance, this can come in oral forms, injections, rings, patches, implants, and insertions.

- Insulin – usually used to manage diabetes mellitus Type I or Type II; this can come in many formulations from ultrashort acting to long-acting. All of which could affect weight.

- Neurologic medications – often used for seizure and memory disorders, fibromyalgia, and other chronic pain syndromes; include such drugs as Depakote, Diazepam, and Memantine.

2. Do weight loss medications work?
   - In my practice, I use them a lot, sometimes pharmaceutical and sometimes nutraceutical (premium quality pharmaceutical grade) supplements. I find most people will need some method of appetite control, even when they don't think they have an appetite problem. The appetite has to be managed in order to get full engagement and compliance for other areas of the weight loss process. Because the appetite is driven by brain and gut hormones primarily, these are the types of appetite control meds

I use, those targeted to those central stations.

- To ensure maximum safety and results, it's very important for the physician prescribing weight loss medications to be well-versed and have in-depth knowledge of the proper use of these medications, or else the efforts can prove to be futile. Selecting the appropriate weight loss medication is dependent upon a number of things, from coexisting medical conditions to concurrent medication use to types of appetite patterns displayed.

- Medication duration depends upon several factors: efficacy, side effects, tolerability, and prescribing guidelines from the manufacturer and/or other regulatory bodies. Some medications are recommended for short-term use, some for long-term use, and some for intermittent use. Sometimes, they may be used slightly longer under certain circumstances, documented by the physician.

- While some may experience weight gain off of medications, that doesn't necessarily indicate a dependency. Dependency on weight loss medication in the clinical sense is not likely; however, many people do feel more in control of their eating when they are able to use the medications when needed.

Selection, initiation, management, and treatment using medications should be handled only by experienced professionals. I can't stress this enough. Just because someone can prescribe you medications doesn't necessarily mean they should prescribe them. Beware of drive-thru pill mills and bootleg, too-good-to-be-true offers. If it seems too good to be true, it probably is too good to be true. Use caution, do your research, and carefully select anyone who will be helping you with your weight loss goals. Ask for credentials, background, training, experience, and references from one, three, and five years prior.

Girl, Get Ready! Lesson #18:

Just because someone can prescribe something doesn't mean they should, and getting a second opinion is okay as well.

Action Step #18:

Make a list of all your medications. What purpose or condition do you take them for and what side effects should you be aware of?

19

Motivation: I Need Help

Be your own hype man.

One thing I've found to be true is that transformation is not for the weary or faint of heart. No matter how badly we desire to be successful at anything, especially weight control, enthusiasm can quickly fade at the faintest glimpse of defeat. Even when things are going well, it can be hard to maintain kick-butt fervor to keep charging ahead full steam. That's not a surprise nor a condemnation; that's a human condition that is widely studied in human psychology around performance.

According to Olya Bullard, a professor at University of Winnipeg, there are two motivational systems operating in every human being. The first system, called promotion, focuses on rewards. The second system, called prevention, focuses on punishment.

As for promotion, reward systems are a common way to cultivate lasting intensity toward making a goal. In our office, we give a buck per pound that can be applied toward future services. That seems to keep the client engaged by celebrating every pound lost. It's a clear way to see the progress made from ground zero. But as people pass the midpoint toward their goals, something happens, says Bullard, who conducted her research with Rajesh V. Manchanda of the University of Manitoba. They stop focusing on how far they have come and start focusing on how far they have to go. The prevention system kicks in. As people contemplate their distance from the end point, they concentrate more on the chances they won't reach it and the negative consequences if they fail to do so.

Overcoming waning eagerness may require framing new goals or creating new ways of encouraging by discouraging. What does that mean? It means stating to clients to lose five more pounds this month versus don't stop losing, you're closer than you think, whatever you do, don't gain a pound next week. You may have done that for yourself or someone you know, not realizing you were actually practicing such tactics.

The truth is, motivation is most effective when it comes from within. In other words, self-motivation packs the most powerful punch. Courage, passion, purpose, and willingness are the four cornerstones of igniting the power within, making you unstoppable in your quest.

Now, outside encouragement can be useful to get you over a hump and can definitely help keep us on the right path. However, relying on external accolades, acknowledgments, ego boosts, and the approval of others can lead to a dead end, leaving you stuck, afraid, and uncertain about the future. Whenever complacency, fear, or lack of clarity hang out, you can be on the lookout for a dip in drive and likely a crawl backward, meaning the wrong direction.

I can think of countless clients who are what I term "ready, ready," and they are unstoppable. They follow every recommendation, they are coachable, positive, and goal-oriented, and they anticipate results no matter what. Those are generally my star players, and I look forward to the journey of exclaiming what they've already decided will be true. On the contrary, I can also think of the majority of clients who start out skeptical, with reservations and hopes that things will "work out this time." I'm eager to work with this client as well, yet I know the pace will be slow and steady as we will need to remain vigilant and flexible to keep the momentum along the way. Both will eventually reach their goals; it's just the difference between flying versus driving a minivan. There's more to look out for on the scenic route traveled in the minivan, whereas the flight will only take off, fly high in the clouds, and land.

I usually keep my clients involved with two-way communication, software programs that provide alerts, and frequent check-ins to reinforce plans and progress. Again, I suggest working with a team when engaging weight loss and establishing clear mile markers to keep the end in plain sight.

Girl, Get Ready! Lesson #19:

Motivation is an inside job.

Action Step #19:

Think of the three biggest accomplishments you've made in your life so far. Then, for each accomplishment, write down one thing that motivated you to achieve that goal. Be specific and honest. Notate which ones were intrinsic or internally driven and those influenced by an external factor or for someone else's benefit. Now, use that to create your go-to list of self-motivators. Give the list to the person closest to you, or who knows you best. Ask them to refer to this list when you need a reminder or a pick-me-up to stay the course.

20

Maintenance: This Is the Hardest Part

The same thing it takes to get there it takes to stay there.

I love watching people reach their goals! The look of pride and joy on their faces is unforgettable. Fortunately, I get to witness this elation often as my clients meet the final milestone they worked so diligently to reach. In my office, we have even incorporated an end of the program celebration, which includes a before and after photo, a certificate of achievement, and an induction into the REALity Stars Club. In the midst of all the high fives and fist pumps, I know, and intuitively they know, this is not the end.

As with most things, there's a journey then a destination then another journey awaiting your next adventure. Sometimes, we really do want to see things as D-O-N-E with a big, green checkmark beside it, but it doesn't work that way altogether, especially with weight loss. The purpose of including this chapter is not to instill fear or incite dismay. The point is to reinforce what may be obvious to some and not so obvious to others. This is the part where we talk about semantics. Go to www.girlgetreadybook.com for a more detailed explanation.

Weight Loss	Weight Management	Weight Control
• Active Phase • Passive Phase	• Prevention • Maintenance Strategies	• Boundaries • Empowerment

Although commonly used interchangeably, "weight loss," "weight management," and "weight control" are different terms. We should spend a little time explaining how these concepts differ and why they matter in your long-term success. In my practice, weight loss is a very dynamic process. I explain to new clients that their weight loss process will happen in phases and stages. The first of those I categorize as active weight loss phase and passive weight loss phase. In the active phase, we are going full-court press to stimulate the metabolism to release stored fat that has been chilling out in its dormant state in conservation mode. That stored fat is then actively converted to free fatty acids and glycerol molecules that can be easily used by the muscles and other organs for energy to keep your body functioning. The more fat we pull out of storage, the smaller the numbers on your scale. Ideally, in its most profitable state, the numbers decrease a little each day. Even if it's not daily but continues to decline consistently, we have entered the active weight loss zone. We like that, and we like to stay there as long as possible to reach the end goal.

Passive weight loss is generally what follows the active phase. In this state, there's nothing particularly special or intense that's being done, but the balance of energy available to energy used over time accumulates on the energy used side day after day and week after week, such that weight loss happens gradually by following a consistent daily routine that includes healthy food choices, productive physical activity, and an emotional and personal environment that is supportive of a well-functioning metabolism. All in all, the metabolism, the lifestyle, the energy balance, and the environment are all working toward the release, use, and loss of excess fat. In general, weight loss is predominantly driven by what we eat (or don't eat for that matter) far more than what we do.

Weight management, on the other hand, is a principle of prevention. The overall goal is to keep the weight from going up, focusing on inhibiting weight gain. "One of the best predictors of success in the long-term management of overweight and obesity is the ability to develop and sustain an exercise program" (*Weight Management: State of the Science and Opportunities for Military Programs*, NCBI). One point of caution I make with my patients is that when exercise is incorporated to maintain weight loss, especially early on once the goal weight has been achieved, exercise can actually present as much of a challenge to promote weight gain as it does to prevent weight gain. That's probably as clear as mud. Let me put it this way. When you are successful at losing weight, your hard work and sacrifice are paying off, you have started an exercise routine, and things seem to be going along fine until all of a sudden, your appetite gradually increases, and you begin to snack a little more. You add an extra helping and before you can say Holy Bologna, the numbers on the scale begin to creep up, leaving you frustrated and bewildered. Literally, I've had patients standing with the shrugging shoulders emoji saying WTF! Usually this is someone who plugged their ears during my maintenance spiel, or they became head over heels in love with their new look and the ride into the sunset headed toward oblivion.

What's the maintenance spiel you're probably asking? Of course, there are fancy and complex explanations, but for you, I'll try to keep it simple. When the body has lost weight, it sometimes questions the motive in a benevolent attempt to return to where you were at your previous weight which the body has grown accustomed to as your norm. It determines that it must do things to make you return to that safe and familiar place, not recognizing that the weight loss was intentional and hard work. There's a specific place in the brain called the hypothalamus that helps to maintain the body's internal balance called homeostasis. It functions as the link between the endocrine (hormone) system and the nervous system. In this case, it regulates weight by regulating hormones that govern the feeling of fullness and signals of hunger, sleep cycles, stomach and digestive secretions, body temperature, and more. When this sensitive control center senses danger or imbalance, its defenses kick in to produce hormones that counteract. Even exercise can trigger a protective response, causing a rise in appetite and impede fat release, which underscores the importance of supervision and guidance with weight and food consumption. These have to be balanced before, during, and after the weight loss process to ensure the hypothalamus has "reset" at the new weight and is ready to maintain the new baseline weight. I always remind my clients to let the body learn to maintain, and that's an art as much as it is a science.

Weight control is the bridge between the previous two terms, weight loss and weight management. Being able to accomplish both losing the weight and preventing weight gain is the essence of weight control. Controlling your weight requires you to get in the driver's seat and stick it out no matter what the terrain.

To be in control of your weight requires you to act from a position of personal power. You must bring together the ability to self-direct, self-motivate, and self-sustain your new successful habits. The best way to do this is to establish a collaborative and synergistic flow between the mind, body, and spirit triad. When you are able to create harmony at the core of your existence, the struggle ends and the beautiful, cooperative flow of winning energy begins to manifest. Having now a firm foundation of the mind and body interactions, let us venture ahead to the final frontier—the spirit.

Girl, Get Ready! Lesson #20:

Achieving success is one thing but maintaining success requires another level of motivation.

Action Step #20:

Using magazine photos or other inspiration pieces, create a lifestyle board divided into four quadrants: nutrition, physical activity, stress, and social outlets. In those four areas of your life, design a winning game plan to maintain your results. For a detailed example, visit www.girlgetreadybook.com.

Spirit

21

What Does That Word Really Mean?

Your spirit is your guide, so take good care of it.

I purposely saved this section for last. Why? Because I needed you to see and process the science, biology, and psychology of understanding how the body works for, and at times, seemingly against you. As consumers, we have been conditioned to accept, embrace, and believe in what is known, needing proof that our arguments are validated. As a physician and a scientist, I, too, find it completely natural to question, hypothesize, analyze, test, and make conclusions based on human theory developed within human ability.

However, I have found room in all of my scientific, practical reality to activate the spiritual power within to elevate my life beyond levels that could be explained by logic or reason alone. As a spirit-led personal success coach, I have been trained, gifted, and found purpose in the ability to do the same for others. I don't profess to be devoutly endowed or well-versed in the historical accounts of religious deity. I'm not ordained or licensed to preach to the masses. I don't run away from those who are nor do I debate the uncertainties of philosophical or personal opinions. I'm putting in a lot of disclaimers here in an effort to let you know the next several chapters are not placed here to root for or against any religion or belief system.

My personal persuasion is that there is an infinite and sovereign God who is all-knowing, all-powerful, and all-loving who is the Creator and overseer of this vast world. The good news is you don't have to agree or disagree to relate to the next several chapters. Trust me—that's not necessary nor is it the point. While I identify with the Christian faith, attend a multicultural, multiethnic church with a global reach, love praise and worship music, and teach my children the power of prayer, it doesn't commit you to any of the above in order to relate to the nine principles we are about to explore. I would assert these have universal applications. My intention is to simply convey that separate from affiliations, we are all spiritual beings.

Girl, Get Ready! Lesson #21:

We are all connected to the universe and have the ability to draw upon this extraordinary association to realize our dreams, manifest miracles, and witness wondrous acts in our lives and in the earth.

Action Step #21:

Time to plug God into your spiritual GPS
Track how God has delivered in your life. Recall a time something amazing or miraculous, lifesaving or life changing happened that you knew was a divine intervention.

22

Where We Go Wrong in the Spirituality Discussion

Wake up your spirit; it needs you.

In spirituality, we often go wrong in four common ways:

1. Having one-size-fits-all approaches to how we experience the world of spiritual existence – In part, this happens in the context of religion, which starts out from the very beginning as a separatist mindset fostering an us-versus-them approach. Most religions, I would argue, speak of love and togetherness as core principles. It's funny (well not really funny) how that only holds true if you happen to be in the same religious belief system. If you aren't, then it's frowned upon. In fact, in some faiths, you are considered wrong for socializing, dating, or marrying someone outside your religion, despite the fact that love and togetherness in those instances are the basis of those relationships. When we expect everyone to believe and behave the same, we lose the ability to see the depth and the breadth of the differences in the universe and the respect to honor them.

2. Relying too heavily on religion – Pitting religions against one another based on differences can hardly be a progressive way of encouraging people to explore their own spirituality, meaning their own personal spirit. There is a saying that maintains people can be so heavenly that they are no earthly good. What makes this relevant is when we interpret religious texts in ways that allow us to make excuses or become irresponsible for how our lives turn out because we have too narrow a view of how to apply the principles to our individual lives. On the other hand, we can take text and bend it in our favor to support the things we want to do, even if we know they aren't what's best for us. It's almost like religion has taken the place of decency, intuition, and energetic collaboration with the universe. There are answers within us. We should trust that.

3. Lacking a clear role in spiritual growth – So often, if you are unchurched or not heavily involved in church fellowship, growing spiritually may sound like trying to learn Mandarin without instruction. Sounds pretty unlikely that would happen; it's not impossible, but it would certainly require some serious self-motivation and commitment to do so. Likewise, when it comes to spiritual growth, it takes the exact same to develop a spiritual proficiency that you can rely on for guidance and direction.

When it comes to spiritual clarity and growth, you must

    a. Learn your spirit

    b. Understand your spirit

    c. Challenge your spirit

    d. Probe your spirit

    e. Identify with your spirit

    f. Own your spirit

    g. Respect your spirit

    h. Protect your spirit

    i. Trust your spirit

4. Leaving your spiritual connection up to chance – A common mistake so many people make is going through life as if developing a solid spiritual sense is an involuntary function like breathing. It's not. You have to intentionally and voluntarily put effort into exploring your spiritual DNA. Because your spirit is one of a kind, it's up to you to own up to that and to put actions and practices in place to strengthen your spiritual core, just like you would your abs or glutes. As a distinction from spiritual growth, which refers to internal wiring, spiritual connection is best described as the external wiring that links us with other living beings.

This is the part where we may find that we always seem to hook up with the "wrong guy" or say things like "she and

I never could get along." Nobody ever understands me, I fall too easily, I'm always the backup, I can never find true friends—all of those are a result of poor spiritual connections, and believe it or not, that is your problem, not theirs. It's so easy to place the blame on these people who can't or don't deliver what we expect. Do me a favor and stop it! Do yourself a favor and start owning your inability to make strong and supportive connections. It's all on you. All of it. Yes. I said what I said. Keep reading and you will find out why.

Girl, Get Ready! Lesson #22:

Don't be afraid to explore spirituality for yourself. Though we are often born into our assigned religion, our personal spiritual journey evolves over our lifetime.

Action Step #22:

Time to level up the God in you!
Look at those four points in this chapter. Pick one that you most closely identify with. Examine the origin of that identity.

23

How Does the Spirit Part of Us Work?

Without our spirits, we're just robots.

We neglect to acknowledge that our individual spirit is really an immortal existence that we all embody, which connects us to a Higher Power. This allows us as individuals to use the richness of that connection to enhance our own personal power, which is otherwise limited to our own human ability. It is used to supply unlimited surges of what we know, do, and feel in the tactile world around us. Without divine power, we can only stay at a level that is within our own capacity to effect change in ourselves and the ordinary world around us.

The benefits of tapping into the universal higher power of God is that you now activate limitless, extraordinary abilities and possibilities that you could never facilitate or even imagine on your own. It's like you get to have superpowers that are turned on when your spiritual energy fields magnetize from anywhere and everywhere the energy sensors of God give you access to as a part of the spiritual agreement. It's like being plugged into a universal switchboard. Who wouldn't want that hookup? I know I do. When I first started digging deeper to establish a closer, more nurturing relationship with God, it felt uncomfortable to suggest that

I could just feel and think and trust that God shows up outside of the usual boxed-in costume that is often etched in our minds.

I wanted to know how the spirit of God shows up on Earth whether in my goals, in my decisions and choices, in my surroundings, in my health, in my finances, in my relationships, and in life in general. I became a student of the spirit realm and discovered there was a whole world of experience that I was naturally operating within, and there was so much more to learn about how I could actively engage and even influence what happens in my life, rather than being an innocent bystander, passively standing on the sidelines with my fingers crossed, hoping and praying that my life would just turn out good. Operating that way always felt a little unstable and chancy. Admittedly at times, I can be a bit of a control freak, but that wasn't it. It seemed more like I had this wait-and-see kind of M.O., hanging on the edge of my seat in a what-happens-next position versus taking the lead in my process, harnessing the freedom to choose and the power to create what I truly wanted in my life. Once I began to practice this way of being, the grips of fear and despair began to loosen, and I traded those feelings for peace and hope.

Girl, Get Ready! Lesson #23:

Become your own spiritual boss who serves as the director, manager, leader, and commander of your goals. With divine guidance and your follow through, you are in the zone.

Action Step #23:

Time to become your own spiritual boss.

Write a job description for your spiritual boss position. Outline the position details such as roles and responsibilities, minimal requirements, and general qualifications. Hire yourself for the job. Do a monthly performance review. For an example, go to www.girlgetreadybook.com.

24

How Does the Spirit Relate to Weight Loss?

*Your energy is not just for physical movement,
it causes spiritual momentum.*

Understanding and utilizing the spiritual connection to your inner desires, growth, and abilities is like taking a ski lift up the mountain to reach your dreams and goals. I see patients all the time who are able to get the weight off physically and begin to see other areas of their lives that they aren't as satisfied with as they thought they were because their biggest area of dissatisfaction was their weight . . . or so they thought. By the same token, I have seen the exact opposite, in which case, my patients who achieve success in losing weight become more "enlightened." They begin to see from a whole new perspective and notice they have more freedom, greater life goals, and feel empowered to tap into other areas of their lives that have the potential for greater satisfaction and fulfillment. Most commonly these become most apparent in the areas of relationships, career, and social well-being, the things that tend to be most associated with going beyond surviving and opening the gateway to thriving. I call this developing a sense of spiritual prosperity.

One client comes to mind. She had been through a series of bad long-term relationships, and at a glance, she looked like she had been put through the emotional ringer. She had done all she could to please others her whole life but never seemed to get the same in return. When I began working with her, she could hardly tell me her favorite color without referencing the color her ex-husband liked on her, the color she wore that got the most compliments, or the color car she bought because she got a good deal. The simple question was, "What is YOUR favorite color?" Over the next several weeks of coaching, we discovered that she had no idea of her true identity, she had operated out of old experiences from childhood and early adulthood, and from there, she spent the better part of her life operating from a "pseudo identity." We began to work on creating her own sense of self-identity, so that she could begin to choose for herself what her future would become.

One of her goals was to weigh in at her goal date, which was June 30th. She lost nearly fifty pounds, obtaining her goal two weeks shy of her four-month goal. She went from a size fourteen to a size four without surgery or fad diets. The weight loss was what she came for, but what she gained was far beyond what she could imagine for herself. She gained a real self-identity, became powerful in her own life course, built self-confidence, and established a new sense of self-worth. That success was made possible because through her coaching, she learned to rewire her spiritual connections, create a new lifestyle, and step into a new way of thinking, speaking, living, and being.

Out of this newly defined self, she made plans to travel abroad, adopt a baby girl, and has already begun to reinvent her once toxic, dark, cold home into a warm, secure, and peaceful sanctuary. All of that came from her tapping into her highest self and her connection to the great potential and purpose for her life. The weight was essentially a symptom, not the problem.

Another client—let's call her CJ—was quite the opposite. Well, not entirely opposite. In this case, when CJ came to me, she was 130 pounds overweight, tipping the scale at 280 pounds on her five foot, four inch frame. Despite her long-standing dissatisfaction with her weight, CJ was absolutely gorgeous and seemingly had it all. She had been married to her high school sweetheart for close to twenty years, her husband had a great job that provided a worry-free lifestyle, and she was a stay-at-home mom, raising their school-aged son and daughter. They lived in a nice, five bedroom home in a gated community, had good friends, the whole nine.

After a few visits, she came in looking like a shell of a person, with sunken, dark eyes and barely speaking above a whisper. Clearly something had gone very wrong since her visit one week prior. As she weighed in, tears began to slowly slide down her flushed cheeks, although she had lost three pounds and met her weekly goal. Once we closed the exam room door, she sat on the table facing the empty wall.

I pointedly asked, "What the heck is going on?" At that moment, she deeply inhaled what seemed to be her last breath and softly exhaled, "He's leaving me. He sat across from me at dinner last night and told me he's not happy and doesn't want to be married to me anymore." Her moist, expressionless face told the story of a once well-kept woman now forced to recalibrate her future at the buzzer. We managed to get through the appointment and end on a relatively positive note. She solemnly confirmed in that visit to stay on track and committed to herself no matter what. And that she did.

Each visit she continued to show progress. Physically she was, as they say, "killing the game." She had found a strong sense of survival that kept her forward-moving despite the fact her life had been turned upside down. I began to see her weight loss results become consistent as well as her emotional recovery. Several months passed, and one day she sent a photo of herself, which bore witness to her serious commitment. She looked amazing! Not only had she lost a bunch of weight, but her wide smile and glowing eyes told a far different story from her fairly recent upset. In the photo was a guy who was smiling just as big. I didn't ask outright, but I wondered to myself, who is this guy who's all smiles? I later found out it was her would-be ex-husband, except they had reconciled and were now going stronger than before.

She lost 105 pounds and got down to 175 pounds, a size she had not been since before the birth of her first child fifteen years ago. She was quite proud of her accomplishment and so was I. I had lost track of her for a few months, when during one of our wellness check-in calls, she answered and admitted she was struggling emotionally. Not fully understanding how she could be doing so well with her weight loss transformation and still feel so miserable inside, she had become frustrated and depressed. Old patterns were starting to seep back in. Her spirit was unsettled, her mind followed that lead, and if left unaddressed, her physical self would soon trail along in a downward spiral.

These examples are similar in several ways; however, the outcomes are polarized. Either way, what each of these examples demonstrates is clear: regardless of what the scale says, it's imperative to address the other things that weigh us down in order to optimize both health and happiness.

Girl, Get Ready! Lesson #24:

One of the most critical principles of weight loss, optimal health, and personal success is spiritual alignment.

Action Step #24:

Before you go to bed each night, realign your spirit with your health goals. Say this simple prayer:

Tonight, before I close my eyes to sleep, I release any faults of the day and fears for tomorrow. I hold no grudges or judgments against myself. Each day, I get to decide my course for health and happiness. I commit to making choices that support those decisions. I have the spiritual ability to govern myself accordingly. I have the power to co-create whatever I deeply desire. I couple my actions with my words and my words with my thoughts to manifest what God has already made available to me.

25

Being in Alignment

A weight problem is an alignment problem.

The stories you read in the last chapter are the sort of stories that I've observed for decades in my career as a physician, coach, friend, and even in my own personal life where being in alignment with your true and highest self can make all the difference in the world when it comes to life's goals, plans, and experiences.

The big question whizzing through your mind right this moment must be, what exactly is alignment? I think the best way to answer that question is by starting with what alignment is NOT.

Being in alignment doesn't necessarily mean that everything is 110 percent perfect in your life. It does not mean you never have a care in the world. Nor does it mean you get to skip to the front of the line in everything you do. No, that's not at all what I want to imply here. While being in alignment is certainly a path to success, it doesn't exempt you from having to deal with hard crap in life. An aligned life is not a perfect life. It is a purposeful life.

This is such an important life principle that it's well worth spending a little time here to go back to the fundamentals. Let's start by breaking down the root word of "align," a verb that has a French and Latin derivation meaning "to arrange things in a line, to reduce to a line," and the transitive or reflexive sense of the word means "to fall in line." The noun, "alignment," is defined as "arrangement in a line." So, here you can see the process of aligning is an action using the basic grammatical standard that a noun is a person, place, or thing. It's clearly established that being in alignment is a thing.

Being aligned or in alignment symbolizes the manifestation of three positions:

1. The beginning

2. The middle

3. The end

Neither one of these positions is any more or less or necessary than the other. Maybe you've heard it said before, usually with a very motivating enthusiasm: "It's not how you start, but it's how you finish." While I have even convincingly recited that myself a time or two, though encouraging for sure, this statement can be a bit simplistic. In all actuality, it's far more progressive to know that it's all about the how, what, when, and especially why you start and end and everything in between. In other words, when we are in alignment, we can expect that things will emerge and evolve from three key places: intentions, purpose, and timing. New ideas, opportunities, friendships, breakups, layoffs, promotions, fitness, health, and wellness all relate to those three interactions.

Intentions are the what of alignment. This defines what you desire to accomplish when you are setting out to do something. In this case, this is an important part of making decisions, which guide choices we make in the pursuit of that which we desire. I have this hierarchy I use when coaching clients to create their dream life:

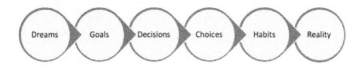

Using this as a guide, the first part is what you want. Once clear, the pathway to achievement is paved in what demonstrates the driving force of alignment.

Purpose is the next step toward alignment. This is an extremely critical part because purpose is the why. I believe this concept is probably the hardest for most people to grasp because we are so busy grinding, hustling, and making moves that we don't always know why we are doing all that we are doing. Purpose is the fuel that is used to make dreams come true. If you understand and commit to your why first, it becomes a superpower when the day-to-day stuff gets really hard. When a tough decision comes up and you can refer back to your why, your purpose, you can navigate that space a lot better.

I remember one of my clients, and at the time, she was a thirty-seven-year-old pediatric nurse who had recently gotten engaged to a great guy she met through a friend a few years ago. They hit it off right away, and they knew within months of their first date that they were destined to be together. He had been married and had two teen sons. The one thing she knew well before they began seriously dating was that she wanted to have kids as soon as she got married. She had already seen a fertility specialist before they even met to explore her options to preserve her ability to have kids someday. She made plans to freeze her eggs but was surprised by what she was told that cold, rainy March day. She would never forget the day the tall, bearded specialist walked in the room, holding an iPad clipped to a yellow chart that he softly laid on the desk in front of her, explaining that the blood work showed several hormone abnormalities that could prevent her from becoming pregnant. She would not be able to have kids if that was not resolved. She described a warm sensation searing through her body and stopping at her throat, which felt like she had swallowed a tennis ball. The room fell silent, and to her, it seemed as if she had been stuffed into a tiny, dark coffin. A tear warmed her cheek, and a hand pressing on her stiff, left shoulder summoned her back to the reality of her physical surroundings. She described zoning out at the very words "not have kids," sending her into a frenzy of worry and despair within minutes of contemplating this awful possibility.

She left the brightly lit office with a two-week follow-up appointment to discuss her options. Those two weeks were agonizing. She pondered the thought of life without kids. Often she would lose her train of thought while at work, wondering, "How can I bear to take care of kids but never have kids of my own?" When she finally returned to see the specialist, after reviewing all of the results, one lasting phrase she recalls and shared in our first visit was, "If you lose weight, you will significantly increase your chances of having children." That was all she needed to spark a ray of hope and get into action. She had struggled with her weight for years. She knew her weight was an issue and somewhat gave up on the notion of shedding those unwanted pounds. This time she vowed it would be different; she would find a weight loss specialist who would help her conquer the weight thing once and for all. She was more determined than ever to win the war and the battle over her weight.

After six months of working together, she had lost over forty pounds, she was feeling great, and more importantly, she was feeling so much better about herself. We were able to go deeper into her past success and failures in weight loss and in life. Through coaching, we identified areas in her life where she gave over her power out of fear, guilt, and shame. We etched out a blueprint for losing the weight, renewing her sense of self-determination and putting her in charge of her life's destiny. Imagine the surprise on the doctor's face when she returned for her appointment three dress sizes smaller and far happier than when they last met. He reviewed her recent lab work and was shocked at the difference from earlier in the year. He pointedly asked her what she had done to lose the weight. She eagerly replied, "I found my purpose for losing it."

Timing is everything. Smack dab in the middle of everything is timing. There's no way to talk alignment without the foundation of timing our life flow. Our mortal clocks tick a little differently than the conventional idea of twenty-four hours a day, seven days a week, 365 days a year. In aligned living, it's not so much about the temporal relationship to how time passes during our life flow that matters most. What aligned timing really becomes is a matter of our own readiness, spiritual availability, and personal responsibility.

> *Growth is never by mere chance; it is the result*
> *of forces working together.*

—James Cash Penney

If you are really ready to move mountains and go forward faster, let your highest self rise up, so that your mind, body, and spirit get on the same page. In other words, line up and head in the same direction at the same time with the same intensity and watch the magic happen! The key here is your highest self! That's the true self that functions with awareness, authenticity, and wisdom. In Deepak Chopra's *Abundance Meditation* series, he refers to a Sanskrit mantra that defines this as: existence, consciousness, and bliss.

Wow! Doesn't that say it all? If we can be in those three places all at once, what might we accomplish? It may seem like a bit of high-level gibberish, but like success, alignment leaves clues. Unfortunately, in our society, most of us are too busy scurrying about what we call life to even slow down enough to check the pulse of existence, eluding consciousness, and allowing material things to define our bliss. In his book, the *Seven Spiritual Laws of Success*, he describes consciousness as our spiritual essence, unbounded, limitless, joyful, pure knowledge, infinite silence, perfect balance, invincible, simplicity and bliss.

The human body is so interconnected to your spiritual essence that you can literally use your body's functioning as a gauge at any moment in time to assess your alignment. The brain, heart, and gut are the most vocal organs that will tell you exactly where you are if you can learn to listen.

Girl, Get Ready! Lesson #25:

Where there is alignment there is:
Clarity, peace, joy, awareness, intuition, discernment, wisdom, creativity, passion, happiness, hope, ease, freedom, purpose, willingness, sensing, knowing, ingenuity, expansion, abundance, prosperity, and love.

Action Step #25:

Carefully examine that list and use your body's reaction or state of being when you were doing something or made a decision that wasn't really in alignment with your true self. Did you feel confused? Unsettled? Guilty? Frustrated?

26

Clear Purpose

Self-love is different from self-like.

Do you clearly know your purpose? Most people don't. They have an idea of what they do or have done and assume that it's related directly to their career or vocation. It would be far too easy and a bit narrow-minded for us to believe our purpose is so singular. Now, don't get me wrong, I believe our occupations can and are certainly, in part, an outlet to demonstrate our purpose, yet by no means is that it. But because we spend so much of our time and energy working, we can sometimes feel that we're living out our life's purpose.

As much as I would like to keep it simple, which I believe is true, I believe in some ways defining one's purpose is equally complex. I'm by no means going to suggest I have it all figured out; philosophers have had this decidedly unresolved discussion for a very long time. Here's what I do believe about purpose:

- It is as <u>unique</u> as a person's fingerprints.
- It is a <u>divine</u> assignment.
- It is <u>dynamic</u> and <u>changes </u>over our lifetime.
- It is largely for the benefit of <u>others</u>, though we reap the blessings as well.
- It is <u>expansive</u> and bigger than what we can imagine.
- It is<u> universal</u>, and we all have one.

I believe the best way to become clear on your purpose is to ask the Creator, which we all can do. I don't think we get to decide entirely, but I believe we get to agree or disagree to live out our purpose as it is revealed to us.

In coaching, I believe it's essential to develop clarity around purpose because I believe it gives us reason, and humans like to know these things. There is a formula I have developed that helps to get us closer to discovering and developing clarity around purpose.

$$\frac{(Talents + Abilities + Gifts)}{Passion} \times Experience = Purpose$$

This is something that can be done and repeated over our lifespan. Clarity of purpose can provide a roadmap to success in every area of our lives, and much like other concepts in the section, keep us on track when life takes off in a whole different direction than what we planned.

As we saw in the earlier example, a clear purpose motivates us to keep going through the hard stuff in life because we know getting to the other side is too important to abandon the mission.

Girl, Get Ready! Lesson #26:

Hope is an anchor when life leaves you shipwrecked. If you know you have purpose, you can make it through anything.

Action Step #26:

Use the formula above to see how closely it reveals or supports your thoughts about your purpose.

27

Love

Only you and God know your purpose.

One of my favorite authors, Gabrielle Bernstein, in her international bestselling book, *Miracles Now*, proposed that in our humanity we engage our world from one of two positions: fear and love. Throughout the book, she gives countless examples of how we go through life filtering between the two. The young author, a highly acclaimed spiritual thought leader and self- proclaimed spiritual junkie, submits that we are often distracted by fear, which prevents us from operating out of our truest nature: L-O-V-E.

In general, the word love brings to mind a feeling, emotion, or experience. But have you ever stopped to think of love as a form of spiritual currency? I have. A number of years ago, I had this wild idea. What if the world didn't have money or any other form of currency, and all we could use to exchange for goods or services is love? How would that change the way we think, make choices, and exist? Would we buy more stuff or less? Would some of us starve to death because we couldn't conjure up enough love to buy even our most basic needs, or would the people with the greatest ability to love and generate love be willing to give that to others, so they, too, could learn to be wealthy? I know it sounds like a sci-fi movie, but it is one of those things that makes you go, "humm."

The need to be loved is one of the most basic human needs, according to Abraham Maslow, a human psychology theorist and creator of Maslow's Hierarchy of Needs. Love, of course, is one of those things we've tried to give a single definition to for years, and the definition here is not up for debate. The point here is more about the need to give, receive, and feel loved over the lifespan from infancy through adulthood.

The ability of a person to give love comes out of the bank of love received first, and then out of the fountain of love felt. Many people are scared and stifled in their ability to generate love because of past hurts, loss, grief, and disappointment. With each of those unhealed wounds, the love capacity gets smaller and smaller. Generating love means that you can give or share love freely, and out of that exchange, love is returned from many sources and can then be received and recycled to flow abundantly within, and then goes back out into the universe and multiplies among living beings.

I commonly find in my work that love is as foreign a concept as life in outer space. This is especially true when it comes to self-love. I recognize that now more than ever, we're seeing articles, blogs, shows, and books about self-love. Do you ever stop to wonder why such a topic must even exist? Like why do we need to specifically point out, coach, and guide people toward loving themselves? It almost seems borderline oxymoronic. I think about that catch phrase from a few years back, "Duh." Why must one be taught to love themselves? Isn't that a given?

The sad reality is that it is not a given. I would have to write a whole other book to go deeper into that point, and maybe I will. But for now, let's talk about how self-love or the lack thereof can impact your personal success goals, especially weight control.

Cathay, a beautifully talented, marketing executive and business owner, enjoyed a lucrative career that brought in multiple six-figures, allowing her to live in a high-end, three bedroom midtown penthouse apartment with Fancy, her fluffy white toy poodle, adorned with pink bows to match her tiny pink toenails, and enjoyed the finer things in life her entire adult life after graduating from a prominent HBCU fifteen years prior. She owned real estate property in her Louisiana hometown, had sorority sisters to hang out with, and could travel the world, and she did, often on business. In fact, when I met Cathay, she wanted to lose thirty pounds before going on vacation to Fregate Island, Seychelles, in four months to the date of our consultation.

I inquired more about the island and said without thinking, "Wow! That seems like a nice romantic trip in the making." She softly replied back, "I wish. Well, I used to." I quickly realized I should have been more careful in my assumptions and tried to cover it up by saying, "Well, the fact that you're heading to a gorgeous island I've never even heard of is enough to be excited about, Sis. Let's get you ready to have the time of your life." Boy, did I underestimate the depth of that one faux pas.

Cathay decided to work with me, and I began to understand how that statement came about. I learned that Cathay had been engaged to be married to a professional athlete; she had fallen in love at first sight during a business meeting several years prior. She was working on sealing the deal on an account that she had been courting for six months. Cathay, naturally charismatic, found the challenge invigorating and expected to make this client hers for sure. She nailed the deal and got to work closely with her soon-to-be fiancé for most of his off-season, in preparation for a big brand launch. The launch was a great success, and her company was riding high and was the buzz of the athletic marketing industry. The relationship became public after the launch, and the two made quite the couple for about a year.

Then things changed. He was traded to another team, took a pay cut, and played half the time he was accustomed to. He began to find fault in things that she did and began to blame her for all of his problems. She tried everything to make him happy and to feel better about the new changes in his career. Nothing she said or did was ever good enough. She started avoiding him at times to keep from making him angry. He started hanging out more, and things began to spiral out of control. One day, they got into a huge argument, and he called her names she couldn't imagine him ever thinking or, even worse, saying. He left that night and never returned. She fell into a deep depression and had no one to call. She felt so ashamed, alone, and hopeless. She attempted to take her life, and three days later was in a psychiatric hospital unit recovering from a near-miss overdose. She was in therapy and had been started on medications, which she attributed to the onset of the weight gain. She was feeling better overall but now couldn't stand to look at herself in the mirror, having never been that size in her life. The trip was a solo trip to reconnect with herself and push the reset button on her life just in time for her thirty-fifth birthday.

I knew it was crucial for her not only to get back to her old self but to become even better than her old self. Many of her successes were lackluster moments in time because she never felt good enough, always expected more of herself, and seldom felt content let alone proud. She had adapted some compensatory behaviors that were unhealthy although quite admirable from the outside. We discovered that much of her decisions in life were out of fear, not love. And certainly not self-love. She had long ago stripped herself of that after being abandoned by her father when she was nine years old.

Though Cathay has been through years of therapy off and on since college, she had never really gotten past the recurring hurt. Despite being able to dominate professionally, she always felt clueless on how to fix her personal life. We did a coaching and weight loss intensive program. For weeks, we had several sessions and even out-of-office excursions and trust exercises to break through at her core. She had built up so many defenses, it was no wonder therapy had only been marginally beneficial.

She lost the weight, got a new wardrobe, and got a new lease on life. She enjoyed the solo trip, and when she came back, she had lots of pictures of tours and sunrises and sunsets. She seemed to be refreshed and encouraged. I shared with her candidly that I honestly wanted to see her get better before her trip because secretly I worried that she may attempt to take her life again while alone on the island. She chuckled and looked down as she twisted the diamond studded platinum charm bracelet on her left wrist. "Doc, you really amaze me. It was my plan to walk out into the deep, dark ocean at midnight on my birthday."

Cathay decided to continue life coaching with me, although she had reached her weight loss goal. She admitted she was better and had decided on her trip that she wanted to live and she wanted to experience the self-love I had been talking about in our sessions.

When one generates love of self, it stimulates the infinite cycle of giving and receiving as an expression of adoration. It's a sense of soulful connection and personal well-being that is exemplified by appreciation, respect, kindness, intentionality, priority, caregiving, optimal health, worth, value, esteem, confidence, trust, forgiveness, protection, and celebration.

Girl, Get Ready! Lesson #27:

Self-love is irrefutably necessary to be your absolute best. Self-like is equally as important and, at its peak, leads to better self-care.

What's the difference? Self-like is what most people call self-care. They like to treat themselves to nice things, but that is only a small aspect of self-love. Self-love is a vibe that's deep, mature, complete, and unshakeable.

Action Step #27:

Write yourself a love song. Write the lyrics like your favorite artist is going to record it and dedicate it to you. Become your own biggest fan.

28

Lean in to Discipline

Discipline will get you further than willpower.

Discipline is for adults too. Although the meaning has a harsh association with punishment or correction, more proactively, discipline means to instruct, teach, or train. Most of us feel we may have outgrown the notion; however, we should continue to embrace discipline as a lifelong principle that continues to refine who we are and who we become over time.

In the spiritual sense, discipline is the practice of self-control that allows us to benefit from that which is best for us and avoid that which is not. Self-control is an act of love for ourselves that won't stand for compromise when it comes to our best interest. One of the biggest things I've seen my weight loss patients struggle with is discipline.

One of my clients, Arianna, who I had been working with for over a year off and on, had decided it was time to get serious and finally lose the weight once and for all. She had been successful in the past with shedding nearly thirty pounds but had slowly watched the scale creep up again to nearly 200 pounds, her highest weight ever. During the process of more in-depth coaching, we discovered her mindset was centered on a set of temporary changes to her diet that would result in weight loss, and finally, she would reach her destination. With that way of thinking, she built in the thinking that "I only have to do this for a certain period of time to get the weight off, then I can go back to what I really like to eat and live happily ever after."

I challenged her to re-examine her approach. An astute businesswoman and successful serial entrepreneur, I asked her to consider what it takes to build the empire. It takes even more of that to keep the empire. To make it even more plain, we looked at the habits of those she referred to as her "thin friends." As we carefully broke down the things she observed when around them, she began to describe a common theme among them. Her friend, Carmen, five feet and eight inches tall, curly, black hair, and scattered freckles was known in their circle as the Blue Jeans Queen. She never met a pair of jeans that didn't accentuate her long, lean legs and curvy hips, considered her favorite assets on her 143-pound frame.

Whether on a summer getaway or girls' night out, they could count on three things that Carmen had done in the last twenty-four hours: 1) worked out for an hour 2) slept well for at least eight hours 3) ate five fruits and vegetables.

Her bestie, Gina, had maintained her size six physique for over seventeen years, despite having two kids, a set of twelve-year-old twin girls. They always joked at the table that Gina was "the picky one." She always asked the server at least six questions about items on the menu. One common one was, "Is this made in house or prepackaged?" Gina's commitment was that she didn't eat processed food and only ate wild-caught seafood, and on top of that, she never ever ate dessert. No matter how often the crew would laugh at her, calling her a food snob, she never gave it a second thought. Gina downright didn't care. Having several family members who were overweight and had diabetes and high blood pressure, Gina took great pride in her body, her skin, and her health.

Then, there was Sam, a former model and now stylist to the stars, known for having the perfect body. Sam had adopted a vegan lifestyle in her late twenties after she left her modeling career behind in New York City for a simpler way of life down South ten years ago. Sam had suffered with endometriosis and uterine fibroids and decided to change her lifestyle to manage this debilitating and painful condition. Sometimes they would go places that didn't have very many vegan options, yet Sam would find something that would fit, though it was no match for the savory delicious foods they were consuming all around her. Sometimes, Sam wouldn't eat at all, often having eaten before she met up with them, knowing choices are typically unpredictable.

Once we went through these stories, and I even shared a few of my own, Arianna began to see the theme was discipline. They had all made a personal agreement to themselves that would not be compromised no matter what circumstances presented. There were clear and defined non-negotiables, a principle we began to coach on to set the tone for self-control and lasting results.

I teach non-negotiables to all of my clients. Whether it's weight loss or integrity, we all have something that we stand firm on; it's that which I am unwilling to bulge in no matter what. There is very little if anything that would be worth it. Defining non-negotiables is an extremely personal thing. I never suggest what those should be for anyone, but we drill down to what they are based on, the purpose they will serve, and the value they provide when upheld.

Since that time, Arianna was able to establish her own non-negotiables and reframe her way of thinking about a lifestyle that kept her at a healthy and confident weight. She realized that her "thin friends" had not been given free passes and worked at being thin. She, too, would have to work at it, become disciplined, and establish a practice of self-control.

Girl, Get Ready! Lesson #28:

Hard work is not to be confused with discipline. Discipline actually makes the work easier.

Action Step #28:

Ask yourself, what are your non-negotiables? Write them down. If you don't have any, create at least one.

29

The Fulfilled Life

Manifest what you desire, deserve, and dream.

Passionate living is a setup for a fulfilled and joyful life. Passions are often described as doing what you love. People who follow their passions are more likely to have a brighter outlook on life and seek a life that is meaningful. When this happens, there is a greater sense of overall satisfaction and that nothing is missing. This abundant mindset and outlook can significantly influence other areas of life as well. A strong sense of personal well-being stemming from a place of happiness and contentment that is driven by choice breeds a sense of certainty and clarity.

I've found this to be an important indicator of success for patients who lose weight, become healthier, and pursue the things in life that are connected to their true and highest self with even more fervor. One example that comes to mind is a forty-six-year-old father of two daughters. He had gained over 100 pounds while working in a highly stressful job, spending long hours at work and at home on a job he didn't really enjoy. He became so consumed with work, he hardly paid attention to the gradual weight gain or the fact that he was losing precious time with his family.

When I met with him, I discovered that his kids would ask him to do things he no longer could physically do nor had the time to do. He couldn't ride roller coasters with them for years due to his weight. He eventually stopped going with his wife and daughters because he couldn't join in the fun. One thing I knew for sure was that he was passionate about his beautiful girls, and being a great dad was the most important thing in the world to him. He literally beamed with pride at the mention of their names. I could tell that passion would carry him a long way. And it did. He was able to lose nearly eighty pounds and rode roller coasters with his two girls for the first time ever. Ironically, he recalled the exhilarating excitement he once enjoyed, going to amusement parks when he was a young boy, feeling young and vibrant again.

Fulfillment is the achievement of something desired, promised, or predicted. Leading a fulfilled life is not a luxury or lofty ideal. It's the standard for living.

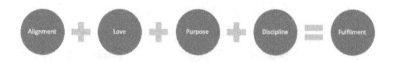

When the energy vibrating around and within are full expressions of each part of that formula, then we maximize the fulfillment available to us.

Girl, Get Ready! Lesson #29:

Living an abundant and fulfilled life is God's plan for us.

Action Step #29:

Time to fulfill your dreams and destiny!
List ten aspects of your life that you are just tolerating.

30

What Can I Do to Enhance My Spiritual Life?

Give yourself permission to be great.

Some things we talked about in the beginning of the book are great ways to enhance your spiritual life. But the first step is to examine your life in general, in a very honest and open way. These are things that we can do to tap into the wellspring of our spiritual core:

- Attend a class on spiritual growth
- Read books
- Listen to podcasts from spiritual thought leaders
- Hire a spiritual life coach, energy healer, or both
- Pray aloud
- Start to practice meditation for clarity
- Take silent walks outside or go to a silent retreat center
- Write letters to God to generate gratitude, clarity, hope, guidance, creativity, or whatever you want or need
- Disconnect from social media for thirty days (or more)
- Start a garden (a container garden on your patio or porch is good if you don't have a yard)

- Write a book about your life story even if you don't publish it

EXPLORING YOUR SPIRITUAL GIFTS

Knowing that you have innate abilities and natural interests can be a great way to tap into your higher self and higher calling. Studies show that people are a lot more satisfied with life when they volunteer and make a contribution to causes bigger than themselves. Very often we can look at our strengths and talents and use those to help others in ways that make a difference in the world.

Gifts can be a way of assuring yourself that you are special and have a reason you've been put on Earth. Sometimes, this reassurance causes us to be more motivated, goal-oriented, and successful in general. One thing I caution is that people can get self-critical and say they don't have gifts and talents mainly because they come so naturally. They think it's not a big deal or anyone can do this or that. I always remind them and myself, that we have to give ourselves more credit and get accustomed to celebrating our abilities.

In my experience, with my weight loss clients, when they are using their gifts and talents, they are happier, more optimistic, and more fulfilled. These positive feelings can be the backbone of positive behaviors. This reinforces a healthy, happy lifestyle. Some examples of spiritual gifts are:

- Encouragement
- Leadership
- Helping

- Administrative
- Giving
- Uplifting
- Teaching
- Hospitality

Girl, Get Ready! Lesson #30:

Operating within your abilities is a great way to reassure your sense of self, foster a feeling of belonging, experience growth and self-development.

Action Step #30:

Time to explore your gifts

- Write down four things people ask you to do for them all the time.
- Write down four things you can do with your eyes closed.
- List anything you've learned on your own or taught yourself to do very well.

There is only one you, and you are uniquely created with divine intentions to light up the world during your brief time in existence on this Earth. None of us know exactly how long we have, but we know for sure our lives have purpose, and we're each given individual assignments that only we can carry out. If you don't do it, it won't get done. Don't miss your chance to contribute to humanity because you are out of shape and in poor health in your mind, body, or spirit. It is the best time ever to take to heart the pages of this book and breathe in the refreshing air of transformation.

We need you now more than ever to step into your greatness, take your greatness to the next level, and reach back to help someone else discover their own greatness. If you haven't done so, yet . . .

Girl, get ready!

About the Author

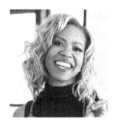

Dr. Jada Moore-Ruffin, widely known as Dr. Jada, is a nationally recognized weight loss specialist, wellness expert, and successful entrepreneur with an award-winning weight loss center. Dr. Jada received her BS degree from Memphis State University and her medical degree from Meharry Medical College, as an honors graduate. She has earned several professional coaching certifications, most notably, integrative nutrition coach and abundant life coach. In addition, she holds double medical board-certifications in family and obesity medicine.

With a passion for weight loss, total wellness, and abundant living, Dr. Jada inspires people to engineer their own happiness, live full out, and create a healthy legacy. She enjoys nature walks, wine tasting, writing, cooking, and volunteering with her beloved sisterhood, Delta Sigma Theta Sorority, Inc.

Dr. Moore-Ruffin resides in Atlanta with her forever husband, Felix. They have three children and a boxer, Oscar. Collectively, they are known as Team Ruffin.

Learn more at www.girlgetreadybook.com

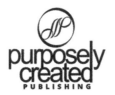

CREATING DISTINCTIVE BOOKS
WITH INTENTIONAL RESULTS

We're a collaborative group of creative masterminds
with a mission to produce high-quality books to position
you for monumental success in the marketplace.

Our professional team of writers, editors, designers,
and marketing strategists work closely together to ensure
that every detail of your book is a clear representation
of the message in your writing.

Want to know more?
Write to us at info@publishyourgift.com
or call (888) 949-6228

Discover great books, exclusive offers, and more at
www.PublishYourGift.com

Connect with us on social media

@publishyourgift